Contents

17th Edition

Antimicrobial Therapy Guide®

Burt R. Meyers, MD, *Editor-in-Chief*
Clinical Professor of Medicine, Division of Infectious Diseases,
Mount Sinai School of Medicine,
and Attending Physician, Mount Sinai Hospital, New York, New York

Contributing Editors

Antonio Anzueto, MD
Professor of Medicine, The University of Texas Health Science Center,
San Antonio, Texas

Thomas M. File Jr., MD, MS
Professor of Internal Medicine, Section of Infectious Diseases,
Northeastern Ohio Universities College of Medicine, Rootstown, Ohio

George A. Pankey, MD
Director, Infectious Disease Research, Ochsner Clinic Foundation,
New Orleans, Louisiana

Jack D. Sobel, MD
Chief, Division of Infectious Diseases, Professor of Internal Medicine,
Detroit Medical Center, Wayne State University School of Medicine,
Detroit, Michigan

Gary P. Wormser, MD
Professor of Medicine and Pharmacology
and Chief, Division of Infectious Diseases, New York Medical College
and Westchester Medical Center in Valhalla, New York.

Published by
Antimicrobial Prescribing, Inc., Newtown, Pennsylvania, USA

This book has been prepared and is presented as a service to the medical community. The information provided reflects the knowledge, experience, and personal opinions of Burt R. Meyers, MD, Clinical Professor of Medicine, Editor-in-Chief, Division of Infectious Diseases, Mount Sinai School of Medicine, and Attending Physician, Mount Sinai Hospital, New York, New York; Antonio Anzueto, MD, Professor of Medicine, The University of Texas Health Science Center, San Antonio, Texas; Thomas M. File Jr., MD, MS, Chief, Infectious Disease Service, and Director of HIV Research, Summa Health System, Akron, Ohio; George A. Pankey, MD, Director, Infectious Disease Research, Ochsner Clinic Foundation, New Orleans, Louisiana; Jack D. Sobel, MD, Chief, Division of Infectious Diseases, Professor of Internal Medicine, Detroit Medical Center, Wayne State University School of Medicine, Detroit, Michigan; and Gary P. Wormser, MD, Professor of Medicine and Pharmacology and Chief, Division of Infectious Diseases, New York Medical College and Westchester Medical Center in Valhalla, New York.

This book is not intended to replace or to be used as a substitute for the complete prescribing information prepared by each manufacturer for each drug. Because of possible variations in drug indications, in dosage information, in newly described toxicities, in drug/drug interactions, and in other items of importance, reference to such complete prescribing information is definitely recommended before any of the drugs discussed are used or prescribed.

International Standard Serial Number: 1520-3352

International Standard Book Number: 1-931981-53-1

Introduction

Burt R. Meyers, MD

Within the past 15 years, a variety of new antibiotics has been introduced for use in clinical practice (eg, β-lactam penicillins, some combined with β-lactamase inhibitors, cephalosporins, and the new macrolides), with carbapenems, monobactams, carbacephems, lipopeptides, and streptogramins being the most recent additions to the antimicrobial armamentarium. In another class are the fluoroquinolones. It is difficult indeed to keep up with both the number and scope of these products if one is not a practicing infectious disease physician. This book is designed as a guide and quick reference to assist in the therapeutic selection of an antimicrobial agent. This manual should supplement, but not substitute for, the prescribing information that is available in the package inserts for all of these agents. Choices of therapy, dosage recommendations, and durations of therapy reflect the collected experience of this author and of other authors who have published their experiences. Obviously, the treating physician must exercise his or her own judgment, taking into account host factors of those who will receive these compounds.

Numerous specific agents are listed, although it is impossible to list, for every situation, all the drugs that are generally considered to be equivalent from a microbiologic standpoint. Some examples of agents regarded as having microbiologic equivalency are noted here: tobramycin, netilmicin, gentamicin, and amikacin (although the last is usually reserved for multiresistant bacteria); amoxicillin and ampicillin (except for shigellosis). Oxacillin and nafcillin have equal efficacy clinically. Piperacillin and mezlocillin are microbiologically equal except that piperacillin is more potent against *Pseudomonas*. The third-generation cephalosporins have some subtle differences but for most organisms are considered equivalent; cefotaxime, ceftizoxime, and ceftriaxone are better for gram-positive organisms, and cefoperazone and ceftazidime for *Pseudomonas*.

Oral agents are available, including a second-generation agent, cefuroxime axetil, and the carbacephems, such as loracarbef. A third-generation agent now available, cefixime, has enhanced gram-negative activity and favorable pharmacokinetics (long half-life) that enable once-a-day dosing. Also available are the fluoroquinolones.

The ideal antimicrobial agent may still be in the future, despite all the knowledge accumulated over the last 60 years. Obviously, we want a safe agent that is able to kill or inhibit pathogens selectively without imposing adverse reactions on the human host. Instead, we often must use agents with a narrow spectrum of activity or agents that too effectively abolish normal protective bacterial flora, predisposing to colonization and infection by opportunistic organisms. Delayed development of resistance would prolong the useful life of an antibiotic. Against this background, as well as the variety of antibiotic choices available, the physician must make a therapeutic selection.

The choice of drug and the duration of therapy reflect the authors' and contributing editors' opinions. New indications for usage as well as toxicities and drug-drug interactions may appear, and it is definitely recommended that, before using or prescribing any drug, the physician consult the latest package insert for complete prescribing information.

The β-Lactam Antibiotics (Penicillins, Cephalosporins, and Carbacephems)

Mode of Action

The β-lactam antibiotics interfere with cell wall synthesis by acting on penicillin-sensitive enzymes, eg, transpeptidases, carboxypeptidases, and endopeptidases, which are found on bacterial cell membranes. These enzymes are believed to be penicillin-binding proteins (PBPs) that interact with the β-lactams and are found on the membranes. PBPs have different physiologic roles, ie, cell configuration, septum formation, and cell lysis. The actual death of cells, or cell lysis, is believed to be caused by active autolytic enzymes. Bacterial resistance to β-lactam antibiotics other than production of β-lactamases may be related to decreased affinities of these molecules to the PBPs or to their inability to penetrate the bacterial cell.

Approach to the Hospitalized Patient

Broad-spectrum antibiotics may be desirable at the initiation of therapy when the causative organism is not known. The third- and fourth-generation cephalosporins and the broad-spectrum penicillins, eg, piperacillin/tazobactam, are active against gram-positive, gram-negative, and anaerobic bacteria. β-Lactam antibiotics are relatively safe compounds and lack ototoxicity and nephrotoxicity associated with aminoglycoside usage. These compounds may be more potent than aminoglycosides in many cases against gram-negative bacilli; many aminoglycoside-resistant strains are sensitive. Because MRSA may be a problem, initial treatment with vancomycin or other agents must be considered.

The approach to a patient with infection of the abdomen or pelvis, where multiple isolates of aerobes and anaerobes are expected, thus could be the use of a newer β-lactam agent rather than two agents (the aminoglycosides and monobactams are not active against anaerobes). Most of these agents have been effective as monotherapy in the treatment of pneumonia, soft-tissue infections, bacteremias, serious urinary tract infection, osteomyelitis, and some in meningitis. Controlled clinical trials have confirmed that single-drug therapy—eg, a new cephalosporin, penicillin, or β-lactam and β-lactamase inhibitor—is equally as effective as some types of combination chemotherapy.

For example, in an elderly patient with either compromised renal function or dehydration, and with suspected sepsis of unknown origin, single-drug therapy is preferred. A new third- or fourth-generation cephalosporin may be selected. MRSA should be covered by other agents.

The use of aztreonam to safely replace aminoglycosides represents a therapeutic modality. This agent should be given with other β-lactams or with clindamycin to cover either gram-positive bacteria or anaerobes. Imipenem/cilastatin and piperacillin/tazobactam represent other alternatives to combination therapy.

The use of preoperative cephalosporin prophylaxis may be responsible for the increase in pseudomonal and enterococcal isolates in the hospital setting. Infection occurring in a patient receiving cephalosporin prophylaxis after abdominal, pelvic, or genitourinary surgery requires an agent that covers *Pseudomonas* and enterococci as well as gram-negative bacilli, organisms that are not within the spectra of the usual prophylactic agents. Piperacillin, cefoperazone, ceftazidime, aztreonam, and imipenem/cilastatin are active against most *P aeruginosa* strains. Review articles on the treatment of gram-negative bacteremia suggest that combination antibiotic therapy is not more effective than single-agent therapy in normal patients. It appears that combination therapy, when the bacteria are sensitive to both agents or when the agents are synergistic, is more effective than monotherapy in immunocompromised, granulocytopenic hosts. Most clinicians believe that bacteremia and pneumonia secondary to *Pseudomonas* are best treated with combination chemotherapy, including a potent antipseudomonal β-lactam and an aminoglycoside or aztreonam in both normal and compromised hosts, although studies have not validated this.

The newer quinolone antibiotics are being used with increased frequency as step-down therapy from parenteral agents in the hospital. This has led to decreased drug costs and, in some cases, shorter hospital stays. Furthermore, their use in the nursing home setting may deter patient transfer to the hospital, thus keeping the patient in a familiar setting and decreasing overall medical costs.

With the use of broad-spectrum agents, an increase in superinfection may occur. Enterococcal, pseudomonal, and *Candida* colonization and superinfection have been reported. Increased use may lead to resistance.

Resistance to β-Lactam Antibiotics

Enzymes

1. β-Lactamases, eg, penicillinases, cephalosporinases. Enzymes found in periplasmic space of gram-negative organisms that hydrolyze β-lactams produce inactive metabolites. Penicillinase is found in the milieu of gram-positive bacteria (*S aureus*). Extended-spectrum β-lactamases (ESBLs) hydrolyze ceftazidime and other third-generation cephalosporins. These β-lactamases are plasmid-mediated enzymes and are found on *Klebsiella* species and *E coli*, etc. There are also inducible β-lactamases found as chromosomal enzymes on many Enterobacteriaceae, including *Serratia*, *Pseudomonas*, *Acinetobacter*, *Citrobacter*, *Enterobacter*, etc. The β-lactam/β-lactamase inhibitor drugs may be active against some ESBL-producing organisms, but not against the inducible cephalosporinases. However, the fourth-generation cefepime is active against many of the chromosomal enzymes and many of the ESBLs. The carbapenems are the most active agents against most β-lactamases. Carbapenemases can deactivate carbapenems.

2. Amylases or amidase remove acyl side chains—of minor importance clinically, but useful commercially in production of semisynthetic derivatives.

3. Esterases, removal of acetyl methoxy function at C-3 (cephalothin or cefotaxime) producing compounds with less antimicrobial activity.

The in vitro hydrolysis of β-lactam antibiotics can be compared by noting enzyme-binding affinities and relative rates of hydrolysis. An antibiotic may be effective against the bacteria that produce β-lactamases, although the compound is hydrolyzable by the extracted cell-free enzyme because penetration into the gram-negative cell, as well as enzyme 'avoidance' or 'flooding' by large concentrations of the β-lactam, may lead to bacterial cell lysis. On the other hand, antibiotics that are β-lactamase stable may induce (derepress) a chromosomally mediated β-lactamase enzyme. The antibiotics may also select for a derepressed mutant; this organism will then continue to make β-lactamases even when the antibiotic is withdrawn. The increase in enzyme may then act as a 'barrier' to the antibiotic, preventing it from reaching PBPs and inhibiting bacterial growth. Another suggestion is that the antibiotic is hydrolyzed by the β-lactamase. Minimum inhibitory concentration (MIC) tube dilution tests or Kirby-Bauer determinations must still be carried out to determine antibiotic sensitivity.

For *S aureus*, however, production of β-lactamase equals resistance to penicillin and ampicillin. While varying rates of hydrolysis may occur for the 'β-lactamase stable' cephalosporins, eg, cefazolin vs cephalothin, these agents are considered resistant to staphylococcal β-lactamases.

4. Combination antimicrobial therapy has been recently introduced, ie, the combination of a penicillin, such as amoxicillin, piperacillin, ampicillin, or ticarcillin, and a β-lactamase inhibitor, such as clavulanic acid, sulbactam, or tazobactam, and has been effective. This combination markedly increases the spectrum of each agent because the inhibitor effectively blocks the β-lactamase enzyme from affecting the antibiotic. Amoxicillin/clavulanate, ticarcillin/clavulanate, ampicillin/sulbactam, and piperacillin/tazobactam are available.

5. MRSA strains produce a new PBP that does not bind the β-lactams, rendering the organisms resistant.

Sequential Antimicrobial Therapy

Rational use of antibiotics to improve quality of patient care while reducing cost must be a goal for clinicians in today's prescribing environment.

The elimination of the need for intravenous access, which is a significant cause of bacteremia, is an important benefit of early switch to oral medication. Reduction in hospital admission time and early discharge are financial benefits. Sequential therapy can also be started in the patient's home with similar advantages.

Many published references have documented the benefits of switch therapy regimens. A multicenter U.S. study of switch therapy involving conversion to oral quinolones such as ciprofloxacin from a number of parenteral regimens revealed projected total savings for drug and hospitalization costs.

Selection of both patient and antimicrobial agent needs to be appropriate in sequential therapy. For example, ciprofloxacin in conjunction with metronidazole is documented as efficacious as switch therapy even in patients with intra-abdominal infections.

New approaches to formerly hospitalized patients have recently been published, eg, shorter oral therapy for acute pyelonephritis and even oral combination therapy for low-risk neutropenic infections.

The Macrolide Antibiotics

Three macrolide antibiotics, with chemical structures related to the prototype macrolide, erythromycin, are available. Clarithromycin, azithromycin, and dirithromycin have a broader spectrum of antimicrobial activity than erythromycin. Clarithromycin and dirithromycin are more active against *S aureus*. Also, these agents have activity against other pathogens. For example, clarithromycin has marked activity against mycobacterial species such as *M avium*, *M chelonae*, and *M fortuitum*. Azithromycin has activity against *Toxoplasma gondii*, *Chlamydia trachomatis*, and the most important respiratory pathogens, including *S pneumoniae*, *M catarrhalis*, *H influenzae*, *C pneumoniae*, *M pneumoniae*, and *L pneumophila*.

In vitro, clarithromycin is also active against *Listeria monocytogenes*. Azithromycin has additional activity against *Neisseria gonorrhoeae*, *Campylobacter jejuni*, and *Bordetella pertussis*. Dirithromycin has additional activity against *L monocytogenes*, *B pertussis*, and *Propionibacterium acnes*.

These three agents have these pharmacokinetic advantages over erythromycin: greater absorption with increased stability in gastric juice, increased tissue penetration, and a longer half-life. The half-life of clarithromycin is approximately 4.3 hours, of azithromycin is approximately 68 hours, and of dirithromycin is 44 hours. All three agents accumulate in large concentrations in neutrophils and other tissues. They have compliance advantages over erythromycin. Azithromycin has approved dosages of 3 days and 5 days, as well as a single one-time dose, depending on the disease. Clarithromycin is taken b.i.d. for 10 days, and dirithromycin is taken once a day for 5 to 14 days.

Clarithromycin and azithromycin have fewer gastrointestinal side effects than erythromycin. Food will decrease azithromycin absorption by 50% when it is taken by capsule, but will increase absorption by 56% when taken by oral suspension. Concomitant antacid may also decrease plasma concentrations of azithromycin. The absorption of dirithromycin is enhanced by food.

These agents have been released for the treatment of selective respiratory tract infections, skin and skin structure infections, and streptococcal pharyngitis; azithromycin is also released for the treatment of nongonococcal urethritis or cervicitis from *C trachomatis*. Dirithromycin is the only macrolide antibiotic with an unqualified FDA approval for *L pneumophila*.

In addition, these drugs have been used in AIDS patients to treat a variety of infections, including *Mycobacterium avium-intracellulare* and toxoplasmosis.

Azithromycin is available in IV, tablet, and oral suspension forms. Clarithromycin and dirithromycin are oral agents.

The package insert should be referred to before using any macrolide concomitantly with any other drugs and to check for new drug/drug interactions.

Mode of Action

Inhibit protein synthesis, 50s ribosome site.

Erythromycin: Bacteriostatic—Activity mostly against gram-positive organisms, also *C diphtheriae* and *M pneumoniae*.

Pharmacology

Erythromycin is a macrolide. Base is acid labile—substitutions minimize dissolutions in gastric acid. Estolate or capsule preparation may give higher plasma levels than stearate or ethylsuccinate with enteric-coated drug. Wide distribution—crosses blood-brain barrier with inflamed meninges, but levels very low. Excretion mainly in bile—only 2%-5% in urine.

Clinical Indications

1. (Group A) β-hemolytic streptococci—as effective as penicillin, alternative to penicillin in treatment and prophylaxis of rheumatic fever in penicillin-allergic patients

2. Pneumococcus—effective alternative to penicillin

3. *Staphylococcus*—if sensitive (not MRSA)

4. *H influenzae*—useful in pediatric therapy, eg, otitis media—combination with sulfonamide for *H influenzae*

5. *Mycoplasma pneumoniae*

6. Pertussis—if therapy indicated, drug of choice

7. Diphtheria—drug of choice

8. Clostridia—effective against tetanus, no effect on toxins. Other clostridia sensitive in vitro

9. Syphilis (primary)—acceptable alternative to penicillin, but requires 30 to 40 g.

10. Legionnaires' disease

11. *Campylobacter* infections

Toxicity and Side Effects

Relatively few—mostly GI distress. Hypersensitivity seen. Candidal superinfection. Hepatotoxicity most serious side effect—abdominal pain, nausea, vomiting, pale stools, dark urine, ulcers, pruritus, hepatomegaly. Abdominal pain believed to be gastritis.

Other Macrolides: In vitro, clarithromycin, azithromycin, and dirithromycin are active against many gram-positive and gram-negative respiratory pathogens, including *S pneumoniae*,

Drug	General Antibacterial Activity	Route	Usual Adult Dosage
erythromycin	gram-positive *M pneumoniae* *Legionella* sp *S pneumoniae* *S pyogenes* some *S aureus* *Chlamydia* *Mycoplasma* *Campylobacter* sp	P.O. IV	250-500 mg q 6 h 1-4 g/d

M catarrhalis, *S pyogenes*, *Mycoplasma* sp, *Legionella* sp, chlamydial isolates, and, to a variable extent, *H influenzae*. These agents are indicated for the treatment of upper and lower respiratory tract infections of mild to moderate severity, skin and skin structure infections, as well as some infections of the genitourinary tract caused by chlamydiae. These compounds have an increased $T^1/_2$ (half-life) compared to erythromycin and are dosed less frequently.

Clarithromycin is approved for these clinical indications: Adults/children: pharyngitis due to *S pyogenes*; acute maxillary sinusitis due to *S pneumoniae*, *H influenzae*, and *M catarrhalis*; uncomplicated skin infections due to *S pyogenes* and *S aureus*; disseminated mycobacterial infection due to *M avium* and *M intracellulare*. Children: acute otitis media due to *S pneumoniae*, *H influenzae,* and *M catarrhalis*. Adults: acute bacterial exacerbations of chronic bronchitis due to *S pneumoniae*, *H influenzae*, and *M catarrhalis*; pneumonia due to *S pneumoniae* and *M pneumoniae*.

Clarithromycin* is contraindicated in patients taking terfenadine or astemizole. Both clarithromycin and azithromycin* are in clinical trials in AIDS patients; azithromycin is also being investigated for the treatment of *Toxoplasma* encephalitis in these patients.

Usual Pediatric Dosage (after 3 mo of age)	Serum Binding %	Serum $T^1/_2$		Some Common Side Effects/Comments
		Normal	Oliguria	
20-50 mg/kg/d given as divided doses q 6 h	18	1.5 h	4-6 h	GI, rash, IV fluid incompatibilities. False SGOT readings. Phlebitis by IV. Available in many forms. Hearing loss rare after IV use. May raise theophylline, warfarin, digoxin, and carbamazepine levels. Contraindicated with use of astemizole, terfenadine, and cisapride.* *S pyogenes* resistance has been reported and up to 20% of group B streptococci may be resistant.

*See package inserts for FDA-approved clinical infections and isolates and other contraindications and drug interactions.

continued on next page

The Macrolide Antibiotics *(continued)*

Drug	General Antibacterial Activity	Route	Usual Adult Dosage
clarithromycin	gram-positive *S aureus* *S pneumoniae* *S pyogenes* gram-negative *H influenzae* *H parainfluenzae* *M catarrhalis* *M pneumoniae* *C pneumoniae* (TWAR) *Legionella** *H pylori*	P.O.	acute exacerbation of chronic bronchitis: ER tab: 2 x 500 mg q 24 h x 7 d** *H pylori* eradication: 500 mg b.i.d. x 10-14 d used in conjunction with other agents: (1) for eradication of *H pylori* to reduce duodenal ulcer recurrence: clarithromycin 500 mg b.i.d. lansoprazole 30 mg q 12 h + 1 g amoxicillin q 12 h x 10-14 d (2) for therapy (triple): clarithromycin 500 mg b.i.d. omeprazole 20 mg + 1 g amoxicillin q 12 h x 10 d (if ulcer presents initially, add 18 d of omeprazole q.d. for healing/relief) (3) for dual therapy: • clarithromycin 500 mg q 8 h + omeprazole 40 mg q.d. (AM) x 14 d. Add 14 d additional omeprazole for ulcer healing • clarithromycin 500 mg q 12 h or q 8 h + 400 mg ranitidine bismuth citrate b.i.d. x 14 d. Add same dose of ranitidine bismuth citrate for 14 d for ulcer relief***

* In vitro activity only.
** Extended-release (ER) tab should be taken with food.
*** Do not use if creatinine clearance is less than 25 mL/min.

1

Usual Pediatric Dosage (after 3 mo of age)	Serum Binding %	Serum T½		Some Common Side Effects/Comments
		Normal	Oliguria	
for children over 6 mo. of age: 15 mg/kg/d divided q 12 h See latest package insert	65	3-7 h	21 h	Fewer GI effects than erythromycin; ventricular arrhythmias are rare; increases theophylline serum. Not approved for pregnant patients. Contraindicated in patients taking terfenadine, astemizole, or cisapride.* Increases carbamazepine levels. Use cautiously in patients with hepatic or renal problems. Dosage adjustment may be necessary. May increase effect of triazolam. May increase digoxin levels. Approved in combination with omeprazole for *H pylori.* Dose of clarithromycin should be halved or dosing interval doubled in patients with creatinine clearance (C_{cr}) <30 mL/min.

*See package inserts for FDA-approved clinical infections and isolates and other contraindications and drug interactions.

continued on next page

The Macrolide Antibiotics *(continued)*

Drug	General Antibacterial Activity	Route	Usual Adult Dosage
clarithromycin *(continued)*	*H pylori*	P.O.	*Mycobacterium avium*: prophylaxis: 500 mg/d b.i.d.* treatment: 750-1,000 mg q.d.-b.i.d. + other agents with activity pharyngitis due to *S pyogenes*: 250 mg q 12 h x 10 d pneumonia: *C pneumoniae*, *M pneumoniae*, and *S pneumoniae*, 2 x 500 mg q.d. x 7 d acute maxillary sinusitis: 500 mg q 12 h x 14 d extended-release (ER) tablet:** 2 x 500 mg q 24 h x 14 d uncomplicated skin infections due to *S aureus*, *S pyogenes*: 250 mg q 12 h x 7-14 d

*If CD4 count is less than 50 cells/mL.
**Extended-release (ER) tab should be taken with food.

Usual Pediatric Dosage (after 3 mo of age)	Serum Binding %	Serum $T\frac{1}{2}$		Some Common Side Effects/Comments
		Normal	Oliguria	
for children over 6 mo. of age: 15 mg/kg/d divided q 12 h See latest package insert	65	3-7 h	21 h	Fewer GI effects than erythromycin; has potential to prolong QTc interval leading to arrhythmias. Should not be used with class I antiarrhythmic drugs (ie, quinidine, procainamide). Increases theophylline serum. Not approved for pregnant patients. Contraindicated in patients taking terfenadine, astemizole, or cisapride.* Increases carbamazepine levels. Use cautiously in patients with hepatic or renal problems. Dosage adjustment may be necessary. May increase effect of triazolam. May increase digoxin levels. Approved in combination with omeprazole for *H pylori*.

*See package inserts for FDA-approved clinical infections and isolates and other contraindications and drug interactions.

continued on next page

The Macrolide Antibiotics *(continued)*

Drug	General Antibacterial Activity	Route	Usual Adult Dosage
azithromycin	*S aureus* *S pyogenes* *S pneumoniae* *H influenzae* *M pneumoniae* *Legionella** *B burgdorferi** *Mycobacterium avium* complex *H ducreyi* *C trachomatis* *N gonorrhoeae* *S agalactiae* *M catarrhalis*** *L pneumophila* *C pneumoniae*	P.O. tablets oral suspension IV	acute exacerbations of chronic bronchitis: 500 mg on first day, then 250 mg/d x 2-5 d as oral therapy or 500 mg q.d. x 3 d community-acquired pneumonia of mild severity: 500 mg on first day, then 250 mg/d x 2-5 d as oral therapy or 2g extended-release (x 1)▲ for those appropriate for oral therapy with community-acquired pneumonia due to *C pneumonia, H influenzae, M pneumoniae, S pneumoniae* acute bacterial sinusitis: 500 mg q.d. x 3 d or 2 g extended-release (x 1) for sinusitis due to *H influenzae, M catarrhalis, S pneumoniae* skin, skin structure infections: 500 mg on first day, then 250 mg/d x 2-5 d as oral therapy tonsillitis*** nongonococcal urethritis: 1,200 mg q week† MAC prophylaxis: 1 g stat

* In vitro activity only.
** Approved for IV.
*** As second-line therapy for tonsillitis.
† If CD4 count is less than 50 cells/μL.
▲ Extended-release oral suspension should be taken without food.

Usual Pediatric Dosage (after 3 mo of age)	Serum Binding %	Serum T½ Normal	Serum T½ Oliguria	Some Common Side Effects/Comments
for children over 6 mo. of age: see latest package insert for community-acquired pneumonia: 10 mg/kg x 1 on day 1 (not to exceed 500 mg/d) followed by 5 mg/kg on days 2 through 5 (not to exceed 250 mg/d) for acute otitis media: 30 mg/kg x 1 dose or 10 mg/kg/d x 3 d in children >6 months	51-7	68 h	unknown	Fewer GI effects than erythromycin. Not approved for pregnant patients. May increase theophylline levels. May interact with terfenadine, cisapride, or astemizole* and should not be used together. However, no clinically significant interactions with theophylline or terfenadine have been reported. Aluminum and magnesium antacids reduce peak levels. Use cautiously in patients with hepatic or renal problems. Dosage adjustment may be necessary. Shorter course therapies enhance compliance.

*See package inserts for FDA-approved clinical infections and isolates and other contraindications and drug interactions.

continued on next page

Drug	General Antibacterial Activity	Route	Usual Adult Dosage
azithromycin *(continued)*			gonococcal urethritis or cervicitis: 2 g stat pelvic inflammatory disease: 500 mg IV q 24 h for 1-2 d followed by 250 mg q.d. P.O. to complete 7 d of therapy hospitalized with commmunity-acquired pneumonia: 500 mg IV q 24 h for at least 2 days followed by 500 mg q.d. P.O. to complete 7-10 d of therapy
dirithromycin	*S pneumoniae* *S pyogenes* *S aureus* *M catarrhalis* *L pneumophila*	P.O.	secondary bacterial infection of acute bronchitis: 500 mg/d x 7 d acute exacerbations of chronic bronchitis: 500 mg/d x 5 d pharyngitis: 500 mg/d x 10 d Pneumonia* due to *S pneumoniae*, *L pneumophila*, or *M pneumoniae*: 500 mg/d x 14 d uncomplicated skin and skin structure infections: 500 mg/d x 5-7 d

* Not indicated for bronchitis or pneumonia due to *H influenzae*; also not indicated for streptococcal skin infections.

Usual Pediatric Dosage (after 3 mo of age)	Serum Binding %	Serum $T½$ Normal	Serum $T½$ Oliguria	Some Common Side Effects/Comments
not indicated	7-51	59 h	—	In patients with either GFR <10 mL/min or impaired hepatic function, use with caution. Nelfinavir significantly increased C_{max} and AUC of azithromycin; thus, close monitoring of side effects (ie, liver enzyme increases and hearing impairment) is warranted. Careful monitoring is recommended when digoxin, ergotamine, cyclosporine, hexobarbital, or phenytoin is used with azithromycin.
not indicated	15-30	8 h (range = 2-36)	unknown	Food enhances absorption. Side effects similar to those experienced with erythromycin. Plasma concentrations of theophylline should be monitored when administered with dirithromycin.* May interact with terfenadine, cisapride, or astemizole* and should not be used together.

*See package inserts for FDA-approved clinical infections and isolates and other contraindications and drug interactions.

The Ketolide Antibiotics

Ketolides are derived from the 14-membered macrolactone ring of erythromycin. They inhibit protein synthesis by binding to the 50S ribosomal subunit. These agents have demonstrated good in vitro activity against many common and atypical/intracellular respiratory pathogens.

Telithromycin is the first ketolide approved for the treatment of acute bacterial sinusitis (ABS), acute bacterial exacerbation of chronic bronchitis (AECB), and mild to moderate community-acquired pneumonia (CAP).

Telithromycin has demonstrated both in vitro and clinical efficacy against *Streptococcus pneumoniae* (regardless

Drug	General Antibacterial Activity	Route	Usual Adult Dosage
telithromycin	gram-positive *S aureus* (erythromycin and methicillin sensitive) *S pneumoniae** gram-negative *H influenzae* *M catarrhalis* *M pneumoniae* *C pneumoniae*	P.O.	for acute exacerbations of chronic bronchitis: 2 x 400 mg q.d. x 5 d for mild to moderate community-acquired pneumonia 2 x 400 mg q.d. x 7-10 d for acute bacterial sinusitis: 2 x 400 mg q.d. x 5 d

*Includes penicillin-resistant *S pneumoniae* and isolates resistant to two or more of the following: penicillin, second-generation cephalosporins, macrolides, tetracycline, and trimethoprim/sulfamethoxazole.

of the presence of macrolide-resistant determinants [*erm*(B), *mef*(A)]), *Staphylococcus aureus* (methicillin- and erythromycin-susceptible isolates only), *Moraxella catarrhalis*, *Haemophilus influenzae*, *Chlamydophila pneumoniae*, and *Mycoplasma pneumoniae*.

The oral bioavailability of telithromycin is unaffected by food. Telithromycin accumulates rapidly and in high concentrations in white blood cells and alveolar macrophages as well as in tissues of the upper and lower respiratory tract, with mean concentrations above the minimum inhibitory concentrations of key respiratory pathogens.

The package insert should be referred to before using any ketolide concomitantly with any other drugs and to check for new drug/drug interactions.

Usual Pediatric Dosage (after 3 mo of age)	Serum Binding %	Serum T½		Some Common Side Effects/Comments
		Normal	Oliguria	
not indicated	60-70	9.8 h	—	Mild to moderate GI effects and visual disturbances (eg, blurred vision). Has potential to prolong QTc interval, which can lead to ventricular arrhythmia, including torsades de pointes. **Not recommended in patients with myasthenia gravis unless no other alternative is available.**

continued on next page

The Ketolide Antibiotics *(continued)*

Drug	General Antibacterial Activity	Route	Usual Adult Dosage
telithromycin *(continued)*	in vitro activity: *L pneumophila*** *S pyogenes***		

**Not FDA approved.

Usual Pediatric Dosage (after 3 mo of age)	Serum Binding %	Serum T½		Some Common Side Effects/Comments
		Normal	Oliguria	
				Avoided in patients who are using class IA (eg, quinidine/ procainamide) or class III (eg, dofetilide) anti-arrhythmic agents or who have congenital prolongation of the QTc interval, hypomagnesemia, hypokalemia, or clinically significant bradycardia. Cisapride should not be used. Levels of midazolam and metoprolol increase when coadministered with telithromycin. Itraconazole and ketoconazole increase levels of telithromycin; but not clinically significant in healthy subjects. Rifampin decreases levels of telithromycin, and concomitant use avoided. Sotalol levels are decreased. Digoxin levels are increased, but no clinical or ECG changes. Food intake does not affect rate or extent of absorption. Simvastatin, lovastatin, and atorvastatin should be stopped while on therapy. May also potentiate effect of oral anticoagulants. Pregnancy: category C.

The Penicillins*

Mode of Action

Interfere with biosynthesis of cell walls of sensitive organisms. Bactericidal. See also 'The β-Lactam Antibiotics' section.

Penicillin G (benzylpenicillin)

Repository forms—procaine and benzathine salts—benzathine produces serum levels for 1 or 2 weeks. Procaine produces high levels, lasts 12 hours. Penicillin is choice for common pyogenic organisms—pneumococci, group A streptococci, sensitive *S viridans*, and meningococci.

Disadvantages:

1. destroyed by penicillinase
2. destroyed by gastric acid
3. allergic reactions

Acid-Resistant Penicillins (Penicillin V)

Oral route, higher level orally than penicillin G. Less active than penicillin G against gram-negative bacteria, *N gonorrhoeae* and *H influenzae*. In most other cases it can be used as oral substitute for penicillin G.

Penicillinase-Resistant Penicillins (PRP)

Injectable

Methicillin: rarely used, oldest acid-labile. Parenteral only. Least protein bound, diffuses into brain, joints, etc. Adequate dosage (6-12 g/d) should be used. Untoward reaction, interstitial nephritis.

Oral and injectable

Oxacillin, cloxacillin, dicloxacillin, nafcillin: Only slight differences in absorption and protein binding—equivalent clinically if adjusted for optimal dosage. Recent increases in methicillin resistance have been reported.

Other Penicillins

Ampicillin: not penicillinase-resistant. Active against *H influenzae* (non-β-lactamase producers), *N meningitidis*, pneumococci, and selected gram-negative organisms—*Salmonella*, *Shigella*, *E coli*, *P mirabilis*.

Bacampicillin: same spectrum as that of ampicillin, but b.i.d. dosage.

Amoxicillin: ampicillin derivative better absorbed, even with food, high blood levels. Bacterial spectrum similar to ampicillin except less active than ampicillin vs *Shigella*. Increasing resistance to *E coli* noted.

Amoxicillin and Potassium Clavulanate: Use of clavulanic acid, a β-lactamase inhibitor, with a penicillin. Clavulanic acid inhibits many chromosomal and plasmid β-lactamases. Clavulanic acid as potassium clavulanate, in combination with amoxicillin, is available in oral form only and is indicated for use in urinary tract infections, soft-tissue infections, sinusitis, lower respiratory tract infections, and otitis media. A new extended-release (XR) formulation is now available, with b.i.d. dosing that achieves higher blood concentration levels.

Ampicillin/Sulbactam: Ampicillin plus β-lactamase inhibitor sulbactam increases spectrum to include β-lactamase-producing *S aureus*, *H influenzae*, *B fragilis*, *M catarrhalis*, *Klebsiella*. Indicated for treatment of intra-abdominal, skin/skin structure, and gynecologic infections.

Piperacillin: Potent broad-spectrum antipseudomonal penicillin. Active against enterococci, *Enterobacter*, *Serratia*, *B fragilis*, and *Acinetobacter*. Resistance to *E coli* increasing. Contains 1.8 mEq Na/g. Use as monotherapy or as synergistic therapy with other agents. Note: ticarcillin, carbenicillin, and piperacillin are susceptible to destruction by staphylococcal β-lactamases and show varying susceptibility to destruction by gram-negative β-lactamases.

Mezlocillin: Similar to piperacillin but less active against most *Pseudomonas* strains than piperacillin.

*Throughout this handbook, ticarcillin is equivalent to carbenicillin, and amoxicillin is equivalent to ampicillin (except for shigellosis).

Ticarcillin/Clavulanate: Ticarcillin plus β-lactamase inhibitor, clavulanic acid, increase spectrum to include *B fragilis*, *S aureus*, *H influenzae*, and *Klebsiella* sp.

Piperacillin/Tazobactam: Piperacillin plus a β-lactamase inhibitor, tazobactam. The most active agent in this class. Active against *Enterococcus*, *Enterobacter*, *Serratia*, *E coli*, *Klebsiella pneumoniae*, *Pseudomonas**, and *Acinetobacter*. Increases piperacillin spectrum to include *S aureus* (MS), *H influenzae* (β-lactamase producing), and *Bacteroides* species, including *B fragilis*.

Carbenicillin: Active against *Pseudomonas*, *Enterobacter* and indole-positive *Proteus*. Not active against *Klebsiella*. High doses needed—400-600 mg/kg/d. Indanyl ester (oral) useful for urinary infections (*Pseudomonas*) only. Oral ester does not produce therapeutic blood levels for systemic infections. Available only in oral form.

Ticarcillin: Active against *Pseudomonas*, *Enterobacter*, and indole-positive *Proteus*, more active than carbenicillin against *Pseudomonas*. Not active against *Klebsiella*.

Amdinocillin: Novel-acting penicillin acting on PBP-2 causing structural changes, ie, ballooning of susceptible strains. Effective against Enterobacteriaceae, including resistant strains. Acts synergistically with other β-lactams but not with aminoglycosides. Not now available in the U.S.

*An aminoglycoside should be added.

Drug	General Antibacterial Activity	Route	Usual Adult Dosage
A. Penicillinase Susceptible			
amoxicillin	similar to ampicillin; less active vs *Shigella*. More active vs *S typhi*, enterococci	P.O.	250-500 mg q 8 h
ampicillin	gram + except *S aureus*; *Shigella*, *Salmonella* including *S typhi*, *E coli*, *H influenzae*, *N gonorrhoeae*, *N meningitidis*, *P mirabilis*	P.O. IM IV	250-1,000 mg q 6 h 0.5-1.0 g q 6 h 1-2 g q 4 h
carbenicillin indanyl sodium	*Pseudomonas*, *E coli*, *P mirabilis* and indole + *Proteus*, *Enterobacter*	P.O.	382-764 mg q 6 h
ticarcillin	same as for carbenicillin	IV	300 mg/kg/d
penicillin G, procaine	group A streptococci *Neisseria*	IM	600,000 U b.i.d.
aqueous crystalline	clostridia pneumococci	IV	1-4 million U q 4-6 h
penicillin G (benzathine)	group A streptococci *Treponema pallidum*	IM	1.2 million U single injection (low, prolonged serum levels); 2.4 million U for syphilis
penicillin V potassium	group A streptococci pneumococci staphylococci (nonpenicillinase)	P.O.	250-500 mg q.i.d.

Usual Pediatric Dosage (after 3 mo of age)	Serum Binding %	Serum T½		Some Common Side Effects/Comments
		Normal	Oliguria	
20-40 mg/kg/d depending on indication	20	1 h	6-18 h	Same as for ampicillin. May cause less GI toxicity.
50-200 mg/kg/d depending on indication	20	1 h	6-18 h	GI symptoms, rash (more common in mononucleosis), anaphylaxis. Renal toxicity rare. *E coli* strains becoming resistant in hospital.
not recommended	50	1.2 h	10-15 h	As above. Use only for urinary tract infections. Approved for prostatitis.
50-300 mg/kg/d	50	1 h	12-17 h	Same as for carbenicillin.
25,000-50,000 U/kg/d (not to exceed adult dosage) — — — IV 25,000-400,000 U/kg/d q 4-6 h	60	6 h by IV, 30 h	–	Anaphylaxis, rash, local reactions, seizures at high doses associated with renal insufficiency.
0.6 mU IM x 1 (<20-27 kg)	—	12 days	12 days	Anaphylaxis, rash, hemolytic anemia, renal toxicity (very rare). Local reactions such as swelling.
25,000-100,000 U/kg/d in 3-6 divided doses	75	1 h	4-10 h	Similar to penicillin G, with minor GI effects.

continued on next page

Drug	General Antibacterial Activity	Route	Usual Adult Dosage
B. Penicillinase Resistant cloxacillin	staphylococci and other gram-positive cocci except enterococci	P.O.	250-500 mg q 6 h
dicloxacillin	as above	P.O.	125-250 mg q 6 h before meals
methicillin	as above	IM IV	1-2 g q 4-6 h
nafcillin	similar to cloxacillin	IV	500 mg-1 g q 4 h
oxacillin	similar to cloxacillin	P.O. IM/IV	0.5-1.0 g q 6 h 1-2 g IV q 4-6 h
piperacillin	*Pseudomonas*, Enterobacteriaceae, *Klebsiella*, enterococci, *B fragilis*, *Serratia*, gram-positive cocci, excluding β-lactamase-producing *S aureus*	IV IM	12-18 g/d, IV (200-300 mg/kg/d) IV divided q 4-6 h 200-300 mg/kg, q 4-6 h 6-8 g/d, IM
mezlocillin	Enterobacteriaceae, *Klebsiella* (enterococci), *B fragilis*, *Serratia*, gram-positive cocci, excluding β-lactamase-producing *S aureus*. Less potent against *Pseudomonas*.	IV IM	12-18 g/d, IV (200-300 mg/kg/d) q 4-6 h 6-8 g/d, IM

1

Usual Pediatric Dosage (after 3 mo of age)	Serum Binding %	Serum T½		Some Common Side Effects/Comments
		Normal	Oliguria	
50-100 mg/kg/d in 4 divided doses	96	0.5 h	1-2 h	Similar to dicloxacillin
12.5-25 mg/kg/d in 4 divided doses	98	0.5 h	1-2 h	Rash, GI upset, eosinophilia, elevated transaminase.
100-200 mg/kg/d	37	0.5 h	4 h	Similar to penicillin G. Also leukopenia, eosinophilia, renal toxicity (interstitial nephritis). No absorption P.O.
25-50 mg/kg/d	90	0.5 h	1-2 h	GI, rash, fever, rare transaminase elevation, anemia, neutropenia. Rare kidney toxicity. High biliary levels.
50-100 mg/kg/d q 4-6 h in divided doses	94	0.5 h	1-2 h	Similar to dicloxacillin. Hepatitis has been described.
studies in progress: data on cystic fibrosis	16	1 h	3-6 h	Broad spectrum. 1.8 mEq Na/g. Toxicity as with other penicillins. Biliary excretion, 20%-25%.
not established	16	1 h	3-6 h	Broad spectrum. 1.8 mEq Na/g. Toxicity as with other penicillins. Biliary excretion, 20%-25%.

continued on next page

Drug	General Antibacterial Activity	Route	Usual Adult Dosage
C. β-Lactams and β-Lactamase Inhibitors ampicillin/ sulbactam	*S pneumoniae* *S pyogenes* *S aureus* *H influenzae*, *M catarrhalis*, *E coli*, *Klebsiella* } β-lactamase producers ± *B fragilis*	IV	1.5-3.0 g q 6 h
amoxicillin/ clavulanate	*S pneumoniae* *S pyogenes* *S aureus* *H influenzae* *M catarrhalis*, *E coli*, *Klebsiella*, *B fragilis* } β-lactamase producers ±	P.O.	250 mg/125 mg q 8 h or 500 mg/125 mg q 12 h or 875 mg/125 mg q 12 h or 500 mg q 8 h for more severe infections
XR-1,000 mg		P.O.	2 x 1,000 mg/62.5 mg q 12 h for acute bacterial sinusitis x 10 d and for community-acquired pneumonia x 7 d
	*S pneumoniae** including intermediate PCN strains *H influenzae*, *M catarrhalis* } β-lactamase producers ±		7-10 d

*Indicated for *S pneumoniae* strains with penicillin MICs of 2 μg/mL or less.

Usual Pediatric Dosage (after 3 mo of age)	Serum Binding %	Serum $T\frac{1}{2}$ Normal	Serum $T\frac{1}{2}$ Oliguria	Some Common Side Effects/Comments
			5-9 h	
For skin/skin structure infections (see package insert for dosing) in children more than 1 yr of age	ampicillin, 28% sulbactam, 38%	ampicillin, 1 h sulbactam, 1 h		Diarrhea 3%, rash 2%, pain at IV site 3%. Though not approved at this time, has role in treatment of outpatient aspiration pneumonia.
40 mg/kg/d (based on amoxicillin component) for sinusitis, otitis media, and lower respiratory tract infections; severe infections; 20 mg/kg/d (based on amoxicillin component) for less serious infections. ES-600: 600 mg amoxicillin, 42.9 mg clavulanate Dose: 45 mg/kg b.i.d. x 10 d for recurrent otitis media XR–not indicated ES-600 mg P.O. ES-600–based on weight 90 mg/kg, divided q 12 h x 10 d	amoxicillin, 20% clavulanic acid, 30%	amoxicillin, 1.3 h clavulanic acid, 1 h	?	May be effective as follow-up to parenteral therapy, and permit shorter hospital stay. Diarrhea greater at higher dosages. XR formulation contraindicated in patients with C_{cr}<30 mL/min and hemodialysis For children with recurrent or persistent AOM due to *S pneumoniae*, *H influenzae*, or *M catarrhalis*

continued on next page

Drug	General Antibacterial Activity	Route	Usual Adult Dosage
C. β-Lactams and β-Lactamase Inhibitors *(continued)*			
ticarcillin/ clavulanate potassium	*S aureus*, other gram-positive bacteria; *Klebsiella* sp, *Proteus* sp *Pseudomonas, E coli, B fragilis*	IV	3.1 g q 4-6 h total daily dose: 12-18 g in divided doses
piperacillin/ tazobactam	*S aureus, E coli, B fragilis K pneumoniae C freundii, P mirabilis M catarrhalis N gonorrhoeae S marcescens*	IV	3.375 g q 6 h 4.5 g q 8 h
	*E aerogenes, E faecalis H influenzae, P aeruginosa**		4.5 g q 6 h or 3.375 g q 4 h for febrile neutropenia**

* An aminoglycoside should be added.
** Not FDA approved, but widely used.

Usual Pediatric Dosage (after 3 mo of age)	Serum Binding %	Serum T½		Some Common Side Effects/Comments
		Normal	Oliguria	
not established	ticarcillin, 45% clavulanate, 9%	ticarcillin, 68 min clavulanate, 61 min	13 h	Broad-spectrum compound monotherapy. Has *S aureus*, *Pseudomonas*, *B fragilis* in spectrum.
not established	20%-23%	1 h	approximately 6 h	Most potent broad-spectrum dual agent with increased activity vs β-lactamase-producing *S aureus*, *B fragilis*, and *H influenzae* strains.

The Cephalosporins

Mode of Action

Inhibition of cell wall synthesis, bactericidal. Stable to staphylococcal β-lactamases.

1. With penicillin-allergic patients, cross-sensitivity occurs in about 19% of cases—**should never be used if patient had anaphylaxis or accelerated allergic reactions unless under the supervision of an allergist familiar with these problems.**
2. Used by some as an alternative to penicillinase-resistant penicillin for hospital staphylococcal infection.
3. Older cephalosporins destroyed by β-lactamase of gram-negatives.
4. May cause false-positive reactions for sugar in the urine.

Older Agents

Active against coliforms, but not active against *Pseudomonas*, *Proteus* (indole +), *Serratia*, *Enterobacter*, or *Acinetobacter*. Less active against *H influenzae* than ampicillin.

Oral Cephalosporins

Cefdinir: A once-daily oral cephalosporin that is highly active against β-lactamase-producing pathogens. Indicated for use in upper and lower respiratory tract infections and skin infections in adults and children. Susceptible pathogens include *S pneumoniae, M catarrhalis, H influenzae, H parainfluenzae, S pyogenes*, and *S aureus*. Available as a capsule and as a pleasant-tasting pediatric suspension.
Ceftibuten: New oral cephalosporin that is highly β-lactamase stable. Offers once-a-day dosing and high bioavailability. Only 3% diarrhea.
Cephalexin: Well absorbed by mouth. Low protein binding. Not deactivated by liver.
Cefaclor: Well absorbed by mouth, metabolized, active against *H influenzae*.
Cefditoren pivoxil: Spectrum similar to other oral cephalosporins.
Cefadroxil: Similar to cephalexin in spectrum, but given b.i.d. or q.d.
Cefixime: A potent, long-acting cephalosporin, allowing once-daily dosing with increased gram-negative spectrum. Highly active against β-lactamase-producing *H influenzae* and *M catarrhalis*.
Cefuroxime axetil: Oral cephalosporin; ester of cefuroxime with same spectrum. Dosing is b.i.d. Indicated for pharyngitis/tonsillitis, otitis media, sinusitis, lower respiratory tract infection, skin/skin structure, and urinary tract infections. A new oral suspension preparation is available. Newly approved for Lyme disease.
Cefpodoxime proxetil: Oral cephalosporin, similar to the second-generation agents. It is indicated for treatment of some respiratory tract infections (pharyngitis and/or tonsillitis) caused by *S pyogenes*; otitis media caused by *S pneumoniae*, *H influenzae* (including β-lactamase-producing strains) or *M catarrhalis*; skin and skin structure infections due to *S pyogenes*; and uncomplicated urinary tract infections (cystitis) due to *E coli*, *K pneumoniae*, *P mirabilis*, or *S saprophyticus*.
Cefprozil: Well-absorbed (95%) compound with activity similar to cefuroxime. Used either b.i.d. or q.d.; available in suspension for pediatric patients. Newly approved for sinusitis.

Parenteral Cephalosporins

Cephalothin: Disadvantages: dose frequency (q 4 h), deacetylation to less active forms by liver (do not use in CSF infection), phlebitis, painful on IM injection. However, much experience allows better standards of use. Most active antistaphylococcal agent.
Cefazolin: Prolonged serum levels, high peak levels, less frequent dosing. High protein binding—useful in prophylaxis.
Cephradine: Not deactivated in liver. Least protein bound in parenteral form.
Cefoxitin: A cephamycin, inhibits gram-positive and gram-negative, aerobic and anaerobic, resistant β-lactamase, induces chromosomally mediated β-

lactamases of some gram-negative bacilli. Does not inhibit *Enterobacter*, *Pseudomonas*, or enterococci; useful in mixed infections. *B fragilis* resistance increasing.

Cefotetan: A long-acting cephamycin derivative with activity similar to other cephamycin derivatives. It has a longer elimination half-life ($T\frac{1}{2}$ is 3.5 h) than has cefoxitin (1 h); it has been administered twice daily in the treatment of mild to moderate infections, including pelvic, intra-abdominal, and postoperative wound infections. Possesses an *N*-methyl thiotetrazole ring, so bleeding due to hypoprothrombinemia may occur.

Cefamandole: IM, IV, *H influenzae*, *Klebsiella*, *E coli*. Possesses an *N*-methyl thiotetrazole ring, so bleeding due to hypoprothrombinemia may occur.

Cefuroxime: IM, IV, *H influenzae*, *Klebsiella*, *E coli*; longer half-life than cefamandole. β-Lactamase stable. Useful in prophylaxis.

Cefonicid: A long-acting parenteral cephalosporin, with a spectrum similar to that of cefazolin. Has advantages of daily dosage. Failures in treatment of *S aureus* endocarditis have been reported.

Third-Generation Cephalosporins

Cefotaxime: Active against gram-positive cocci ($T\frac{1}{2}$ is 1 h). Active in meningitis.

Ceftazidime: β-Lactamase-stable cephalosporin; potent agent against *Pseudomonas* and other gram-negative bacilli; less active against gram-positive (in vitro) and gram-negative anaerobic bacilli. Effective in serious infections, including meningitis.

Ceftizoxime: Spectrum and activity similar to that of cefotaxime, but $T\frac{1}{2}$ is 2 h. May be cost saving with t.i.d. dosage.

Ceftriaxone: β-Lactamase-stable cephalosporin. Active against gram-positive and gram-negative organisms. $T\frac{1}{2}$ is 6-8 h. Central nervous system penetration; can be used in meningitis. May become best prophylactic agent. Long half-life may mean cost savings. Once/day dosing used successfully in serious infections. Useful in home-care therapy. Has been successful in treating late manifestations of Lyme disease, including CNS manifestations and arthritis (preliminary results).

Cefoperazone: Spectrum similar to that of cefotaxime. More potent antipseudomonal agent. Less stable to gram-negative β-lactamases. Biliary excretion prominent. B.i.d. dosing could represent cost saving. Possesses an *N*-methyl thiotetrazole ring, so bleeding due to hypoprothrombinemia may occur.

Fourth-Generation Cephalosporins

Cefepime: A new fourth-generation cephalosporin that appears to be more resistant to β-lactamase hydrolysis. This agent has activity against most gram-positive organisms and most β-lactamase-producing gram-negative bacteria, *Pseudomonas aeruginosa*, including many *Klebsiella pneumoniae* and *Enterobacter* strains that are resistant to ceftazidime.

Other Agents

Carbapenems

Imipenem/cilastatin: Imipenem is a synthetic agent with a broad spectrum of antibacterial activity against gram-positive cocci (excluding methicillin-resistant *S aureus* and *S faecium*), gram-negative bacilli (including *P aeruginosa*, but not *P maltophilia*), and anaerobic organisms (including *B fragilis*). It must be given with cilastatin, an inhibitor of a renal dipeptidase. The half-life of the compound is approximately 1 h. While imipenem is β-lactamase stable, it is a potent inducer of chromosomal type 1 β-lactamase found in many gram-negative bacilli. Seizures have occurred in a subset of patients, and particular caution is necessary in patients with evidence of renal insufficiency. Resistance in *P aeruginosa* strains has been reported.

Meropenem: A parenteral carbapenem with same activity as imipenem (without

the need for cilastatin); has q 8 h dosing.
Ertapenem: A powerful carbapenem with a spectrum similar to imipenem but with poor activity against *P aeruginosa*; 4-hour $T\frac{1}{2}$ allows once-daily dosing.

Aztreonam: A monobactam. Similar spectrum to aminoglycoside. Effective against aminoglycoside- and cephalosporin-resistant gram-negative organisms. Poor activity against gram-positive organisms and anaerobes. Use in penicillin-allergic patients. Low toxicity.

The Cephalosporins

Drug	General Antibacterial Activity (not active against enterococci)	Route	Usual Adult Dosage
A. Oral			
cephalexin	gram-positive: not active vs enterococci (group D streptococci). Gram-negative: active vs *E coli*, *P mirabilis*, *Klebsiella*	P.O.	0.25-0.5 g q 6 h
cephradine	same as cephalexin	P.O.	250-500 mg q 6 h
cefaclor	gram-positive: not active vs enterococci (group D streptococci). Gram-negative: active vs *E coli*, *P mirabilis*, *Klebsiella*, staphylococci	P.O.	0.25-1.0 g q 8 h
cefaclor CD	*S pneumoniae* *H influenzae** *S pyogenes*		Extended-release formulation: 500 mg b.i.d. x 7 d for treatment of acute exacerbations of chronic bronchitis 375 mg b.i.d.x 10 d for treatment of *S pyogenes* pharyngitis
cefadroxil	same as for cephalexin	P.O.	1-2 g/d

*Non-β-lactamase-producing strains

Loracarbef: A new carbacephem antibiotic for oral administration, with in vitro activity against respiratory tract pathogens, including *S pneumoniae, S aureus, S pyogenes*, and, in some indications, β-lactamase-producing *H influenzae* and *M catarrhalis*. Indicated for acute maxillary sinusitis*, otitis media, pharyngitis, bronchitis, pneumonia*, skin infection, uncomplicated pyelonephritis and cystitis due to susceptible strains of indicated organisms.

*Except for β-lactamase-producing *H influenzae* strains

Usual Pediatric Dosage (after 3 mo of age)	Serum Binding %	Serum $T^1/_2$		Some Common Side Effects/Comments
		Normal	Oliguria	
25-100 mg/kg/d	15	1 h	20 h	Rare, but may have rash, eosinophilia. Less active vs staphylococci than parenterals.
25-100 mg/kg/d	15	1 h	20 h	Same side effects as cephalexin.
20-40 mg/kg/d	15	1 h	3 h	Useful in sinusitis. Same side effects as cephalexin.
30 mg/kg/d	20	1 h	20 h	Useful b.i.d. dosage, better compliance. Same side effects as cephalexin.

continued on next page

Drug	General Antibacterial Activity (not active against enterococci)	Route	Usual Adult Dosage
cefixime	*S pyogenes* *S pneumoniae* *H influenzae* β-lactamase ± *M catarrhalis* β-lactamase ± *E coli* *N gonorrhoeae* β-lactamase ± *S marcescens* *Providencia* sp *Citrobacter* sp *P vulgaris*	P.O. tablets oral suspension	400 mg/d or 200 mg b.i.d.
cefuroxime axetil	*S pyogenes* *S pneumoniae* *H influenzae* β-lactamase ± *M catarrhalis* β-lactamase ± *E coli, N gonorrhoeae* *Borrelia burgdorferi*	P.O. tablets oral suspension	250 mg b.i.d. severe infection: 250-500 mg b.i.d. gonorrhea: 1 g x 1 d early Lyme disease: 500 mg b.i.d. x 20 d urinary tract infection: 125-250 mg b.i.d.
cefpodoxime proxetil	*S saprophyticus* *S pneumoniae* *S pyogenes* *E coli* *K pneumoniae* *M catarrhalis* *P mirabilis* *N gonorrhoeae*	P.O. tablets and oral suspension	200 mg x 1 for uncomplicated gonorrhea 100 mg b.i.d. for UTI, pharyngitis and/or tonsillitis 200 mg b.i.d. for community-acquired pneumonia 400 mg b.i.d. for skin and skin structure infections
ceftibuten	*S pyogenes* *S pneumoniae* *H influenzae* β-lactamase ± *M catarrhalis* β-lactamase ±	P.O. capsules oral suspension	400 mg/d

Usual Pediatric Dosage (after 3 mo of age)	Serum Binding %	Serum T½		Some Common Side Effects/Comments
		Normal	Oliguria	
after 6 mo of age: 8 mg/kg/d or 4 mg/kg b.i.d.	65	3-4 h	11.5 h	Once-daily dosing will enhance compliance; potent activity against gram-negative bacteria. Has no significant *S aureus* activity. Highly active vs β-lactamase-producing *H influenzae* and *M catarrhalis*.
tonsillopharyngitis: 20 mg/kg/d divided b.i.d. otitis media and impetigo: 30 mg/kg/d divided b.i.d.	50	1.2 h	10-24 h	Increased absorption if taken after food. New oral suspension available. Newly approved for sinusitis, early Lyme disease, and gonorrhea.
5 mo to 12 years: otitis media (acute): 10 mg/kg/d q 24 h x 10 d maximum: 400 mg/d pharyngitis and/or tonsillitis: 5 mg/kg/dose q 12 h x 5-10 d maximum: 200 mg/d	22-33	2.1 h	mild 3.5 h moderate 5.9 h severe 9.8 h	
>6 mo old: 9 mg/kg/d In pediatric patients, has 70% penetration rate into middle ear fluid.	65	2.4 h		Once-a-day dosing can enhance compliance. Potent activity against gram-negative bacteria; no *S aureus* activity. Highly active in vitro against β-lactamase-producing *H influenzae* and *M catarrhalis*. Only 3% diarrhea in adults.

continued on next page

The Cephalosporins *(continued)*

Drug	General Antibacterial Activity (not active against enterococci)	Route	Usual Adult Dosage
cefprozil	*S aureus* *S pyogenes* *S pneumoniae* *M catarrhalis* β-lactamase ± *H influenzae* β-lactamase ±	P.O. oral suspension	250-500 mg b.i.d.
cefdinir	*S pneumoniae* *H influenzae** *M catarrhalis** *S aureus** *H parainfluenzae** *S pyogenes*	capsules oral suspension	600 mg/d or 300 mg b.i.d.
cefditoren pivoxil	*S pyogenes* *S pneumoniae* *H influenzae* β-lactamase ± *M catarrhalis* β-lactamase ± *E coli* *N gonorrhoeae*	P.O.	400 mg b.i.d. x 10 d for AECB;400 mg b.i.d. x 14 d for CAP; 200 mg b.i.d. x 10 d for pharyngitis and uncomplicated skin/skin structure infections
loracarbef	*S pyogenes,* *S pneumoniae,* *S aureus,* *M catarrhalis* β-lactamase ± *H influenzae* β-lactamase ± *Clostridiu* *Fusobacterium*	P.O. oral suspension	200-400 mg b.i.d.

* Including β-lactamase-producing strains

Usual Pediatric Dosage (after 3 mo of age)	Serum Binding %	Serum T½		Some Common Side Effects/Comments
		Normal	Oliguria	
7.5 mg/kg b.i.d. for pharyngitis/ tonsillitis* 15 mg/kg b.i.d. for otitis media** 20 mg/kg/d for skin and skin structure infections* 7.5-1.5 mg/kg q 12 h for acute sinusitis**	36	1.3 h	5.9 h	Well absorbed (95%). Used either b.i.d. or q.d. Available in suspension form for pediatric patients. Low incidence of GI side effects. Suspension has a pleasant taste for children.
14 mg/kg/d or 7 mg/kg b.i.d.	60-70	1.7		Once-daily dosing enhances compliance. GI side effects observed.
not indicated	88	1-2 h		Same as cephalexin. Not indicated in patients allergic to milk protein. Contraindicated in patients with carnitine deficiency or with inborn errors of metabolism that may cause carnitine deficiency.
7.5 mg/kg b.i.d. for pharyngitis and skin infection 15 mg/kg b.i.d. for otitis media	25	1.1 h	5.6-32 h	Well absorbed, 95%; used either b.i.d. or q.d. Available in suspension form for pediatric patients. Only 1% discontinuation due to GI side effects.

* For patients 2 to 12 years old
** For patients 6 mo to 12 years old

continued on next page

Drug	General Antibacterial Activity (not active against enterococci)	Route	Usual Adult Dosage
B. Parenteral			
cephalothin	gram-positive streptococci and staphylococci; gram-negative *E coli*, *P mirabilis*, *Klebsiella*	IV	0.5-2.0 g q 4-6 h
cefazolin	similar to cephalothin	IM/IV	0.5-2.0 g q 8 h
cephradine	similar to cephalothin	IM/IV	0.5-2.0 g q 4-6 h
cefamandole	adds cephalothin-resistant *E coli*, *Klebsiella*, *H influenzae*	IM/IV	0.5-2.0 g q 4-8 h
ceforanide	similar to 2nd-generation cephalosporins	IM/IV	0.5-1.0 g b.i.d.

1

Usual Pediatric Dosage (after 3 mo of age)	Serum Binding %	Serum T½		Some Common Side Effects/Comments
		Normal	Oliguria	
80-150 mg/kg/d	70	0.5 h	3-8 h	Phlebitis, pain on injection, rash, fever, eosinophilia, leukopenia, elevated transaminase, rare renal toxicity. In serious infections, use 12 g/d. May increase aminoglycoside nephrotoxicity.
25-100 mg/kg/d	85	1.9 h	30-50 h	Phlebitis, raised alkaline phosphatase, elevated transaminase. In serious infections, use 6 g/d. High bile levels. Use in *S aureus* infection is questioned by some.
50-100 mg/kg/d	15	1 h	20 h	Contains 6 mEq Na/g. Rash, eosinophilia, leukopenia, raised transaminase. Pain on injection, some phlebitis.
50-100 mg/kg/d	70	0.6 h	8 h	Has been used as empiric therapy in community-acquired pneumonia.
not known	80	2.9 h	?	Longer-acting 2nd-generation cephalosporin.

continued on next page

Drug	General Antibacterial Activity (not active against enterococci)	Route	Usual Adult Dosage
cefuroxime	*S pyogenes*, *S pneumoniae*, *S aureus*, *E coli*, *Klebsiella* sp, β-lactamase-producing *H influenzae*, *M catarrhalis*. Enters CSF. β-lactamase stable.	IM/IV	0.75-1.5 g q 8 h for life-threatening infections, 1.5 g q 6 h
cefoxitin	adds cephalothin-resistant Enterobacteriaceae and *B fragilis*. Inactive against *Enterobacter* sp.	IM/IV	1.0-2.0 g q 4-8 h
cefotetan	adds cephalothin-resistant Enterobacteriaceae and *B fragilis*. Inactive against *Enterobacter* sp.	IV/IM	• 500 mg-2 g q 12 h IV • 3 g q 12 h IV for life-threatening infection • 1-2 g for prophylaxis before clean contaminated or partially contaminated surgery.
cefonicid	similar to cefazolin, cefamandole	IV/IM	1 g/d (IV or IM); 1 g b.i.d. (IV or IM) or 2 g/d for severe infections

Usual Pediatric Dosage (after 3 mo of age)	Serum Binding %	Serum $T\frac{1}{2}$		Some Common Side Effects/Comments
		Normal	Oliguria	
50-150 mg/kg/d	50	1.3 h	10-24 h	Longer half-life—more stable to β-lactamase than cefamandole. Used in meningitis. Used as empiric therapy in community-acquired pneumonia and surgical prophylaxis.
80-160 mg/kg/d	70	0.6 h	10-18 h	Used in mixed aerobic-anaerobic infections. Can be given IM if mixed with lidocaine.
not established	88	3-4.6 h	10 h	Used in mixed aerobic and anaerobic infections. Useful as prophylactic agent.
not established	90	4.5 h	25 h	Similar to other 2nd-generation cephalosporins; decreased *S aureus* activity.

continued on next page

The Cephalosporins *(continued)*

Drug	General Antibacterial Activity*	Route	Dosage
Third-Generation cefotaxime	gram-positive organisms (except enterococci); *N gonorrhoeae*, GNB, including aminoglycoside-resistant strains; less active against *B fragilis* in vitro	IV IM	1 g b.i.d. for uncomplicated infections 1-2 g q 8 h for moderate to severe infections Up to 12 g/d for life-threatening infections
cefoperazone	gram-positive and gram-negative organisms; potent antipseudomonal cephalosporins; less β-lactamase stable	IV IM	1-2 g b.i.d.; 6-12 g/d in divided doses for severe infections
ceftizoxime	gram-positive and gram-negative (GNB) organisms, β-lactamase stable	IV IM	2 g q 8 h 3-4 g q 8 h IV for life-threatening infections
ceftazidime	β-lactamase stable; potent antipseudomonal cephalosporin—more active against gram-negative organisms than gram-positive in vitro	IM IV	250 mg-2 g q 8-12 h

*Treatment of gram-negative bacteremia in granulocytopenic hosts probably should be with two agents to which bacteria are sensitive and/or synergistic. Gram-negative pneumonia probably requires two agents.

1

Pediatric Dosage	Serum Binding %	Serum T½ Normal	Serum T½ Oliguria	Common Side Effects/ Comments
useful in neonatal and GNB meningitis, and in neonatal and infant infections up to 1 wk: 50 mg/kg q 12 h 1 to 4 wk: 50 mg/kg q 6-8 h	36-50	1.0 h parent 1.8 h metab- olite	—	Monotherapy-amino- glycoside sparing. Useful in meningitis. Partially metabolized to active desacetyl form. Metabo- lite and parent drug act synergistically against some bacteria in vitro.
not established	82-93	2 h	—	Monotherapy-amino- glycoside sparing. Dual route of elimination: hepatobiliary and renal. Less dosage adjustment in renal failure.
not established	30	1.7 h	—	Monotherapy-amino- glycoside sparing. Not metabolized. Excreted virtually unchanged in the urine in 24 h.
neonates: 0-4 weeks 30 mg/kg, IV b.i.d. infants and children 1 mo-12 yr: 30-50 mg/kg, IV q 8 h maximum of 6 g/d in immunocompro- mised and those with cystic fibrosis or meningitis	5	1.8 h	—	Useful in gram-negative meningitis. Low inci- dence of diarrhea. Active against *Pseudomonas*, but less active against gram-positive (in vitro) and gram-negative anaerobic bacilli. β-Lactamase resistance occurs in *Klebsiella* and *Enterobacter* strains.

continued on next page

The Cephalosporins *(continued)*

Drug	General Antibacterial Activity*	Route	Dosage
Third-Generation *(continued)* ceftriaxone	gram-positive organisms, except enterococci, and gram-negative bacilli (GNB), including aminoglycoside-resistant strains; *N gonorrhoeae*. β-Lactamase stable; long $T^1/_2$ of 6-8 h. Once-daily dosage possible. meningitis: 100 mg/kg/d in divided doses; not to exceed 4 g/d.	IM IV	1-2 g/d or 1-2 g b.i.d.
Fourth-Generation cefepime	gram-positive organisms *S pyogenes* *S aureus* *S pneumoniae* *S viridans* gram-negative organisms *Enterobacter* sp *K pneumoniae* *P aeruginosa* *E coli* *P mirabilis*	IV IM	0.5-1 g IV/IM q 12 h x 7-10 d for severe infections: 1-2 g IV q 12 h x 10 d 2 g q 8 h for febrile neutropenia

*Treatment of gram-negative bacteremia in granulocytopenic hosts probably should be with two agents to which bacteria are sensitive and/or synergistic. Gram-negative pneumonia probably requires two agents.

Pediatric Dosage	Serum Binding %	Serum $T\frac{1}{2}$ Normal	Serum $T\frac{1}{2}$ Oliguria	Common Side Effects/ Comments
up to 1 wk: 50 mg/kg q 24 h 1 to 4 wk: 50 mg/kg q 24 h <2 kg 50-75 mg/kg q 24 h >2 kg 50-100 mg/kg/d q 12-24 h not to exceed 4 g/d	95	6-8 h	—	Long half-life; use as preoperative prophylaxis; useful in meningitis; cost saving with once-daily dosing. Preoperative prophylaxis of 1 g for vaginal or abdominal hysterectomy or coronary artery bypass surgery. Repeated dose is not usually required. Has been used to treat late complications of Lyme disease, including CNS manifestations and arthritis.
For pediatric patients up to 40 kg: uncomplicated and complicated urinary tract infections (including pyelonephritis), uncomplicated skin and skin structure infections and pneumonia: 50 mg/kg q 12 h (for febrile neutropenia patients, q 8 h). Maximum dose should not exceed adult dose. See package insert regarding insufficient data to support use in some *H influenzae* type b infections.	20	2 h	13.5 h	Active against many ceftazidime-resistant strains of *K pneumoniae* and *Enterobacter*. Similar side effects as other cephalosporins.

The Monobactams and Carbapenems

Monobactams

Drug	General Antibacterial Activity*	Route	Usual Adult Dosage
aztreonam	gram-negative aerobic bacilli, especially *P aeruginosa*, *Serratia*, *Klebsiella*, *Enterobacter* sp. Anaerobes and gram-positive bacteria are resistant.	IV IM	urinary tract infection: 0.5-1 g q 8 or 12 h moderately severe symptoms: 1-2 g q 8 or 12 h life-threatening: 2 g q 6 or 8 h maximum dose: 8 g/d

Carbapenems

Drug	General Antibacterial Activity*	Route	Usual Adult Dosage
imipenem/ cilastatin	*S pneumoniae* *S viridans* *S aureus, E coli* *H influenzae* *K pneumoniae* *N meningitidis* *P aeruginosa* most resistant gram-negatives *Acinetobacter* sp *Enterobacter* sp anaerobes	IV	500 mg q 6 h

*Treatment of gram-negative bacteremia in granulocytopenic hosts should be with two agents to which bacteria are sensitive and/or synergistic. Gram-negative pneumonia probably requires two agents.

Usual Pediatric Dosage	Serum Binding %	Serum T½		Common Side Effects/ Comments
		Normal	Oliguria	
30 mg/kg q 8 h maximum dose: 120 mg/kg/d	56	1.7 h	4.9-8 h	Gram-negative spectrum similar to aminoglycosides without nephrotoxicity or ototoxicity. Empirically, should be used with other antibiotics to enhance gram-positive/ anaerobic spectrum. Has a role in penicillin-allergic patients. (See warning on package insert.)

Usual Pediatric Dosage	Serum Binding %	Serum T½		Common Side Effects/ Comments
		Normal	Oliguria	
≥3 months of age: recommended dose for non-CNS infections is 15-25 mg/kg q 6 h	20 imipenem 40 cilastatin	1 h	3.4 h imipenem 16 h cilastatin	Broad spectrum of activity. Stable to β-lactamases. Seizures may occur, especially in patients with decreased renal function; therefore, careful dose adjustments are necessary.

continued on next page

The Monobactams and Carbapenems *(continued)*

Carbapenems *(continued)*

Drug	General Antibacterial Activity*	Usual Route	Adult Dosage
meropenem	*S pneumoniae, S viridans* *S aureus, E coli* *H influenzae, K pneumoniae* *N meningitidis* *P aeruginosa* most resistant gram-negatives anaerobes *B fragilis* *Peptostreptococcus* *B thetaiotamicron*	IV	adults with intra-abdominal infection: 1 g q 8 h IV
ertapenem	*S aureus* (not MRSA) *S agalactiae* *S pneumoniae* (penicillin-susceptible only) *S pyogenes* *E coli* *H influenzae* (β-lactamase negative) *M catarrhalis* *Bacteroides* species, including: *B fragilis, B distasonis,* *B ovatus, B thetaiotaomicron,* *B uniformis* *Peptostreptococcus* *Prevotella bivia* *Eubacterium* *Clostridium clostridioforme*	IV IM	complicated intra-abdominal infections: 1 g/d x 5-14 d acute pelvic infections, including postpartum endomyometritis, septic abortion, and post-surgical gynecologic infections: 1 g/d x 3-10 d community-acquired pneumonia: 1 g/d x 10-14 d complicated skin/ skin structure infections: 1 g/d x 7-14 d complicated urinary tract infections, including pyelonephritis: 1 g/d x 10-14 d

*Treatment of gram-negative bacteremia in granulocytopenic hosts should be with two agents to which bacteria are sensitive and/or synergistic. Gram-negative pneumonia probably requires two agents.

Usual Pediatric Dosage	Serum Binding %	Serum $T^1/_2$		Common Side Effects/ Comments
		Normal	Oliguria	
• with intra-abdominal infection: 20 mg/kg q 8 h (if a child is >50 kg, then 1 g q 8 h) • with meningitis: 40 mg/kg q 8 h (penicillin-resistant strains have not been studied). If child is 75 kg, then 2 g q 8 h	2	adults: 1 h children 3 mo to 2 yr: 1.5 h	increased	Has broad spectrum of activity. Stable to β-lactamases. Does not need cilastatin inhibitor for renal dehydropeptidase. May cause fewer seizures than imipenem/cilastatin.
not known	80-90	4 h	increased	Diarrhea 5.5%, nausea 3.1%, headache 2.2%, vaginitis 2.1%, phlebitis 5%. Must decrease dose in patients with creatinine clearance (C_{cr}) <30 mL/min and in patients on hemodialysis. For patients with decreased renal function, see Table 24 in Section 17. No adjustment for hepatic insufficiency.

The Aminoglycosides*

Mode of Action

Inhibit protein biosynthesis; bactericidal.

Factors in Resistance

1. Inactivation of aminoglycosides:
   a. Production of aminoglycoside-inactivating enzymes, ie, adenylating, phosphorylating, hydroxylating enzymes by gram-negative bacilli (GNB).
2. Failure to penetrate bacterial cells. Important resistance mechanism with aminoglycosides, ie, amikacin.

Older Aminoglycosides

Kanamycin, neomycin, streptomycin. Their use is now limited due to increasing resistance and toxicity. Cross-resistance between kanamycin and neomycin complete—partial cross-resistance between kanamycin and streptomycin. None absorbed orally to a significant degree. Distribution good after IM injection. These agents do not enter central nervous system except in neonates. Poorly bound to protein. Excreted by glomerular filtration.

Drug	General Antibacterial Activity	Route	Usual Adult Dosage
gentamicin	GNB, esp. *Pseudomonas* and *Proteus*, *E coli*, *Klebsiella*, *Enterobacter*, *Serratia*. All anaerobes resistant. Pneumococci and streptococci resistant, staphylococci variable	IM IV	1.0-1.7 mg/kg q 8 h Adjust dose according to renal function.
kanamycin	*E coli* *E aerogenes* *Proteus* (not *Pseudomonas*)	IM IV	15 mg/kg/d in 2 doses. Not to exceed 1.5 g/d.
neomycin	*K pneumoniae*, *Proteus*, *E coli*, *E aerogenes*	P.O.	2-3 d in hepatic coma—25 mg/kg q.i.d. x 1 d, then 12.5 mg/kg b.i.d. (4-12 g total daily dose) Use with caution because of potential for ototoxicity/nephrotoxicity. Maximum length of treatment: 2 wk.
spectinomycin**	*N gonorrhoeae*, if penicillin-resistant or in penicillin-allergic patient	IM	2 g single dose.

* Dosage adjustments are required for all aminoglycosides when used in patients with renal insufficiency. Serum levels should be monitored. *In the elderly, the use of a formula based on creatinine clearance, rather than on weight, may be desirable.*

** This compound is an aminocyclital.

Toxicity Includes:
1. auditory and vestibular;
2. neuromuscular block—apnea—especially if used with neuromuscular blocking drugs, rapid IV injection; reversed by use of calcium or neostigmine; and
3. nephrotoxicity—increased with antecedent renal conditions. Toxic effects made more likely by dehydration, loop diuretics, concurrent use of another aminoglycoside, overdosage, elderly subjects, hypotension. Toxicity related to blood levels. Monitor—audiometry, kidney function tests, and serum levels.

Streptomycin: Toxic to vestibular and auditory nerves. Renal toxicity uncommon. Emergence of resistance dictates use of concomitant drug. Shows synergy with penicillin against enterococci—especially for endocarditis. Use in TB with one or more anti-TB drugs. Use in brucellosis, tularemia, plague.

Kanamycin: Use limited by resistance. Newer aminoglycosides (gentamicin, tobramycin) have replaced this agent. Ototoxicity more frequent than with other agents. Also nephrotoxic.

Usual Pediatric Dosage (after 3 mo of age)	Serum Binding %	Serum T½		Some Common Side Effects/Comments
		Normal	Oliguria	
<1 week: 5 mg/kg/d >1 week: 6.0-7.5 mg/kg/d in 3 divided doses	0	2 h	35-50 h	Nephrotoxicity and ototoxicity; use with caution in elderly; monitor serum levels with renal insufficiency; audiograms may be necessary.
15 mg/kg/d	0	2 h	30-50 h	Auditory toxicity, nephrotoxicity, neuromuscular block. Do not use until sensitivity established.
E coli enteropathogenic—50 mg/kg/d in 4 divided doses, oral—2-3 days	0	2 h	50 h	Other agents are preferred. Nephrotoxicity and ototoxicity even when given P.O. Should not be used parenterally.*
—	0	2 h	—	Rash, fever, painful injection. Use 20-gauge needle. Rarely used for disseminated infection. Fails in pharyngeal gonococcal infection.

*Has been used for gut sterilization and bowel preparation prior to colonic surgery. Rarely used as treatment for infection.

continued on next page

The Aminoglycosides* *(continued)*

Neomycin: Oral form; topical application also. Parenteral form very toxic—not used. Despite limited absorption, toxic effects from oral and topical route, if patient has decreased GI motility, renal failure, prolonged widespread topical use. Other toxic effects include allergy, diarrhea, spruelike syndrome (malabsorption). Uses—hepatic coma (bowel disinfection) and preoperative colonic preparation.

Gentamicin: Narrow range between therapeutic and toxic levels—monitoring—renal tests, blood levels. Caution in renal failure—adjust according to actual blood levels rather than algebraic formulas. Synergism with penicillin for enterococcus; with β-lactams for *Pseudomonas*. Use topi-

Drug	General Antibacterial Activity	Route	Usual Adult Dosage
streptomycin	*M tuberculosis, Yersinia, Brucella, Francisella*	IM	1-2 g/d For TB dosage, see anti-TB drug section
amikacin	similar to gentamicin—more effective in resistant species	IM IV	15 mg/kg/d in 2-3 doses (maximum 1.5 g/d)
tobramycin	similar to gentamicin except more active in vitro vs *Pseudomonas*; *Serratia* less sensitive in vitro than to gentamicin	IM IV	1.0-1.7 mg/kg q 8 h Adjust according to renal function. Loading dose in renal failure.
Experimental Aminoglycosides:			
sisomicin	same as gentamicin	IM IV	5 mg/kg/d in 3 doses

*Dosage adjustments are required for all aminoglycosides when used in patients with renal insufficiency. Serum levels should be monitored. *In the elderly, the use of a formula based on creatinine clearance, rather than on weight, may be desirable.*

cally, selects resistant strains. For CNS use intrathecally. Indications—gram-negative bacteremia, urinary tract infection, pulmonary infection, meningitis (intrathecal), burns, bone and joint infections, endocarditis, soft-tissue infections.

Tobramycin: Clinically equivalent to gentamicin. Potent in vitro action against *Pseudomonas*. Active against many gentamicin-resistant *Pseudomonas*. Not active against Enterobacteriaceae resistant to gentamicin.

Amikacin: Kanamycin derivative. Active against most species resistant to gentamicin, kanamycin, tobramycin, and netilmicin. Useful in infections due to resistant bacteria, *Serratia, Pseudomonas,* and *Providencia*.

Spectinomycin: Indicated only for gonorrhea. Use in penicillin resistance or allergy to penicillin. Not bactericidal.

1

Usual Pediatric Dosage (after 3 mo of age)	Serum Binding %	Serum $T_{1/2}$		Some Common Side Effects/Comments
		Normal	Oliguria	
20 mg/kg/d 2 doses	30	2 h	35-50 h	Reserved for use in tuberculosis in combination with isoniazid. Plague, tularemia, brucellosis.
15 mg/kg/d in 2 doses	0	2 h	35-50 h	Ototoxicity. Nephrotoxicity. Similar to gentamicin.
6.0-7.5 mg/kg/d in 3-4 doses	0	2 h	35-50 h	Similar precaution to gentamicin in renal failure.
not approved	0	2 h	35-50 h	Same toxicity as for gentamicin.

The Tetracyclines

Mode of Action

Prevent protein syntheses at the level of the binding of transfer-RNA-amino acid complexes to the ribosomes. Bacteriostatic.

Pharmacology

Incompletely absorbed in the upper GI tract—doxycycline and perhaps minocycline better absorbed and less affected by food. Inactivated by chelate formation with metal ions, eg, calcium, magnesium, ferrous—impaired absorption with milk products, antacids, iron supplements. Different tetracyclines have differing half-lives and concentrations, but all yield therapeutic blood levels. Excreted by kidney—half-life extended in renal failure. Doxycycline not excreted by kidney and has been used in renal failure. Biliary excretion of all agents.

Antimicrobial Spectrum

All tetracyclines active against most gram-positive cocci, excluding group D streptococci (*Enterococcus*), and against many gram-negative bacilli and *Borrelia burgdorferi* (agent of Lyme disease). *Mycoplasma, C pneumoniae,* and *C trachomatis* also inhibited. Some tetracycline HCl-resistant *S aureus* are inhibited by minocycline and doxycycline. Some tetracycline-resistant

Drug	General Antibacterial Activity	Route	Usual Adult Dosage
tetracycline HCl	many gram-positive and gram-negative *Mycoplasma* *Bacteroides* *Rickettsia* *Chlamydia* *Borrelia burgdorferi*	P.O. IV	usual daily dose: 1 to 2 g in 4 equal doses depending on severity of infection
chlortetracycline	as above	P.O. IV	as above
oxytetracycline	as above	IV/IM	250 mg q 24 h or 300 mg/d in 2-3 doses
demeclocycline	as above	P.O.	150 mg q 6 h or 300 mg b.i.d.

Bacteroides inhibited by doxycycline and minocycline.

1. Primary Choice: *Pasteurella, Francisella, Brucella, Vibrio cholerae, M pneumoniae, Rickettsia, Borrelia,* psittacosis/ornithosis agents (*Chlamydia*). Lymphogranuloma venereum agents, trachoma/inclusion conjunctivitis.

2. Effective, but Not Primary Choice: *Pneumococcus*, group A streptococci (10% resistant). Group B streptococci, some *E faecium*, anaerobic streptococci. *Listeria, Bacillus anthracis, E coli* (many strains), *H influenzae, N gonorrhoeae, H ducreyi, Clostridium tetani, C perfringens, T pallidum, Bacteroides* species (subsp *fragilis*).

Resistance to Tetracyclines

E coli and *Shigella* increasingly resistant. Also pneumococci—thus, prescribe only after culture shows sensitivity, eg, urinary tract infections, upper respiratory infections. *Bacteroides* also showing increasing resistance.

Tigecycline, a new glycylcycline, is not affected by two major tetracycline resistance mechanisms: ribosomal protection and efflux. There is no cross-resistance between tigecycline and other antibiotics, and tigecycline is not affected by other resistance mechanisms (eg, β-lactamases, target changes). This drug is also bacteriostatic.

Pediatric Dosage	Serum Binding %	Serum T½		Some Common Side Effects/Comments
		Normal	Oliguria	
not recommended for children	60-70	8.5 h	100 h	GI, allergy, rash, primary dentition discoloration, liver toxicity, elevated CSF pressure (benign) in infants, renal toxicity (increases BUN), photosensitivity. Give 1 h before or 2 h after meals. Do not administer with food, milk, or antacids or to children. Do not give to pregnant patients.
not recommended for children	70-75	5.6 h	11 h	As above
not recommended for children	35	9.6 h	100 h	As above
not recommended for children	90-95	—	—	As above + diabetes insipidus syndrome on long-term therapy.

continued on next page

The Tetracyclines *(continued)*

Drug	General Antibacterial Activity	Route	Usual Adult Dosage
doxycycline	As for tetracycline HCl. More effective against anaerobes. Useful in pelvic inflammatory disease (PID), *Chlamydia* infections, *Borrelia burgdorferi* Active against many strains of vancomycin-resistant *E faecium*	P.O. IV	200 mg on day one, then 100 mg/d
minocycline	As for tetracycline HCl. Useful in carriers of *N meningitidis* (oral only); *Corynebacterium acnes.* Also useful in PID and *Chlamydia* infections. Has been used in Japan for methicillin-resistant *S aureus* (MRSA).	P.O. IV	200 mg initially, then 100 mg b.i.d.
methacycline	as for tetracycline HCl	P.O.	150 mg q 6 h

Pediatric Dosage	Serum Binding %	Serum T½ Normal	Serum T½ Oliguria	Some Common Side Effects/Comments
not recommended for children	90-95	16 h	16 h	Similar to tetracycline HCl; may be administered with food and milk. Avoid exceeding dosage. Less tooth staining. May be used in renal failure. Used as prophylaxis for prevention of traveler's diarrhea. Useful in treatment of PID (see section on gynecologic infections). Has been used to treat multidrug-resistant strains of enterococci.
not recommended for children	75-80	18 h	35 h	As for tetracycline. Vestibular symptoms can be prominent in females especially; less dizziness if given as divided dose q 8 h. Active against many methicillin-resistant *S aureus.*
not recommended for children	90	14 h	100 h	As for tetracycline HCl.

continued on next page

Drug	Antibacterial Activity	Route	Adult Dosage
tigecycline	*S aureus* (including MRSA) *S pyogenes* *S agalactiae* *S anginosus* *E faecalis* (susceptible to vancomycin) *C freundii* *E cloacae* *E coli* *K pneumoniae* *K oxytoca* *B fragilis* *B thetaiotaomicron* *B uniformis* *B vulgatus* *C perfringens* *Peptostreptococcus* VREF* *S epidermidis** *L monocytogenes** *P multocida** *A baumannii** *S marcescens** *Prevotella** *M abscessus** *M chelonae** *M fortuitum**	IV	100 mg IV administered over 30-60 min x 1 dose, then 50 mg q 12 h for 5-14 d Indications: • Complicated intra-abdominal infections due to *E coli, E cloacae, C freundii, K pneumoniae, K oxytoca,* MSSA, *Streptococcus* sp, *B fragilis, C perfringens, Peptostreptococcus* sp • Complicated skin/skin structure infections due to *E coli,* vancomycin-susceptible *E faecalis,* MSSA, MRSA, *Streptococcus* sp, *S pyogenes, B fragilis* **Note:** Dosage with severe hepatic impairment (Child-Pugh C) is 100 mg followed by 25 mg q 12 h.

*Not FDA approved for this organism.

Pediatric	Serum Binding %	Serum T½		Comments
		Normal	Oliguria	
Use in patients under 18 years not recommended	71%-89%	Single-dose study: 27.1 h	Same	Not indicated for *Pseudomonas* spp. No dosage adjustments for renal failure, hemodialysis, race, or gender. Mainly metabolized by liver; not removed by dialysis. Avoid in pregnancy and young children. Use caution if giving to nursing mother. Main side effects are GI in nature: nausea, vomiting, diarrhea.

Clindamycin, Lincomycin

Mode of Action

Inhibits protein synthesis, 50s ribosome site. Bacteriostatic, some bactericidal activity against gram-positive cocci, anaerobic cocci, and bacilli. Not active against *S faecalis* (enterococci); some clostridial species are resistant. Clindamycin more active in vitro. Cross-resistance between lincomycin and clindamycin. Some cross-resistance with erythromycin. Erythromycin antagonizes the lincomycins.

Clinical Pharmacology: Clindamycin or Lincomycin—IV, IM, P.O.

Clindamycin: Indications limited to anaerobic infection (especially *B fragilis*) and severe gram-positive infections.

Drug	General Antibacterial Activity	Route	Usual Adult Dosage
clindamycin	*S pneumoniae* *S pyogenes* *S aureus* anaerobic sp *B fragilis* *Fusobacterium* sp	IM/IV P.O.	150-600 mg q 6 h 150-300 mg q 6 h
lincomycin	gram-positive cocci anaerobes	IM IV P.O.	600 mg q 12-24 h 600 mg q 8-12 h 250-500 mg q 8 h

Use in penicillin-allergic patients.
Lincomycin: Variable oral absorption, better parenterally. Both not significantly protein bound, wide distribution, enters CSF poorly with inflamed meninges. Hepatic excretion.

Toxicity and Side Effects
Diarrhea. Pseudomembranous colitis (PMC) due to overgrowth of *C difficile.* Either metronidazole or vancomycin may be used as therapy of PMC.

Cholestyramine may be helpful since it binds toxin. Do not use antidiarrheals, eg, diphenoxylate, as they may increase toxic effects. Other side effects very uncommon, eg, allergies. Occasional transient liver function test abnormalities. Superinfection not common.

Usual Pediatric Dosage (after 3 mo of age)	Serum Binding %	Serum T½ Normal	Serum T½ Oliguria	Some Common Side Effects/Comments
15-40 mg/kg/d divided q 6-8 h IV	25	2-2.5 h	6-10 h	Better absorbed orally but rarely used. Useful in penicillin-allergic patients with gram-positive infections; 10% of peptostreptococci, 15% of group B streptococci, and up to 30% of clostridial species (other than *C perfringens*) may be resistant. Diarrhea, severe pseudomembranous colitis may occur.
IV— 10-20 mg/kg/d in 2-3 doses	25	2-2.5 h	6-10 h	Popular outside US. Diarrhea, severe pseudomembranous colitis may occur.

The Streptogramins

Drug	General Antibacterial Activity	Route	Usual Adult Dosage
quinupristin/ dalfopristin	A streptogramin antibiotic with activity against gram-positive cocci, including vancomycin-resistant *E faecium* (VREF), *S aureus* MRSA**, GISA*, VRSA* *S pyogenes* *S epidermidis* (including methicillin-resistant strains)* *S agalactiae* *C jeikeium*	IV	complicated skin/skin structure infections: 7.5 mg/kg q 12 h VREF infections: 7.5 mg/kg q 8 h

* In vitro activity only.
** Not FDA-approved for this indication.

Usual Pediatric Dosage (after 3 mo of age)	Serum Binding %	Serum T½		Some Common Side Effects/Comments
		Normal	Oliguria	
not approved	moderate	Q = 3 h D = 1 h	increased AUC	Inflammation and pain at infusion site; rheumatologic syndrome. Inhibits cytochrome P-450 -3A4, and plasma concentrations of drugs metabolized by this enzyme will be increased, including cyclosporine, the antihistamines, antifungals, terfenadine, and anti-HIV drugs (protease inhibitors and NNRTI). See package insert for all possible drug interactions.

The Oxazolidinones

Drug	General Antibacterial Activity	Route	Usual Adult Dosage
linezolid	vancomycin-resistant *E faecium* (VREF) *S aureus* (including MRSA) *S agalactiae* *S pneumoniae* (penicillin-sensitive strains) *S pyogenes** *E faecalis** *S epidermidis** *S hemolyticus** *S pneumoniae** viridans streptococci* *P multocida** *M tuberculosis*** *Nocardia* species** Atypical mycobacteria**	IV P.O.	community-acquired pneumonia due to penicillin-sensitive *S pneumoniae* with bacteremia and *S aureus* (methicillin-sensitive): 600 mg IV or P.O. q 12 h x 10-14 d Nosocomial pneumonia, *S pneumoniae* (penicillin-sensitive) or *S aureus* (including MRSA): 600 mg IV or P.O. q 12 h x 10-14 d complicated skin/ skin structure infections *due to S aureus*, MRSA, *S pyogenes*, *S agalactiae* (not studied in diabetic foot or decubitus ulcers): 600 mg IV or P.O. q 12 h x 10-14 d uncomplicated skin/ skin structure infections, *S aureus* (methicillin-sensitive) and *S pyogenes*: 400 mg IV or P.O. q 12 h x 10-14 d

* In vitro data only.
** Not FDA-approved for these pathogens.

Usual Pediatric Dosage (after 3 mo of age)	Serum Binding %	Serum T½		Some Common Side Effects/Comments
		Normal	Oliguria	
VREF: 10 mg/kg IV or oral q 8 h x 14-28 d >12 yr: 600 mg q 12 h x 14-28 d* nosocomial pneumonia: 10 mg/kg IV or oral q 8 h x 10-14 d up to 11 yr >12 yr: 600 mg q 12 h x 10-14 d complicated skin/skin structure infections: 10 mg/kg IV or oral q 8 h x 10-14 d up to 11 yr >12 yr: 600 mg q 12 h x 10-14 d uncomplicated skin/skin structure infections: <5 yr: 10 mg/kg oral q 8 h x 10-14 d 5-11 yr: 10 mg/kg oral q 12 h x 10-14 d	31	4.5-5 h	4.5-5 h	Because this drug is a monoamine oxidase inhibitor, patients must avoid foods with high tyramine content. Metabolites increase with renal dysfunction. Does not induce the P-450 cytochrome system. Reversible enhancement of pressor response with pseudoephedrine and phenylpropanolamine.

*See package insert for more dosing information.

continued on next page

The Oxazolidinones *(continued)*

Drug	General Antibacterial Activity	Route	Usual Adult Dosage
linezolid *(continued)*	vancomycin-resistant *E faecium* (VREF) *S aureus* (including MRSA) *S agalactiae* *S pneumoniae* (penicillin-sensitive strains) *S pyogenes** *E faecalis** *S epidermidis** *S hemolyticus** *S pneumoniae** viridans streptococci* *P multocida** *M tuberculosis*** *Nocardia* species** Atypical mycobacteria**	IV P.O.	VREF infection, including bacteremia: 600 mg IV or P.O. q 12 h x 14-28 d

* In vitro data only.
** Not FDA-approved for these pathogens.

Usual Pediatric Dosage (after 3 mo of age)	Serum Binding %	Serum $T^{1}/_{2}$		Some Common Side Effects/Comments
		Normal	Oliguria	
community-acquired pneumonia: 10 mg/kg IV or oral q 8 h x 10-14 d neonates: up to 7 d: 10 mg/kg q 12 h after 7 d: 10 mg/kg q 8 h up to 11 yr, then 600 mg q 12 h	31	4.5-5 h	4.5-5 h	**Warning:** Myelosuppression (including anemia, leukopenia, pancytopenia, and thrombocytopenia) has been reported in patients receiving linezolid. In cases where the outcome is known, when linezolid was discontinued, the affected hematologic parameters have risen toward pretreatment levels. Complete blood counts should be monitored weekly in patients who receive linezolid, particularly in those who receive the drug longer than 2 wk, those with preexisting myelosuppression, those receiving concomitant drugs that produce bone marrow suppression, or those with a chronic infection who have received previous or concomitant antibiotic therapy. Discontinuation of therapy with linezolid should be considered in patients who develop or have worsening myelosuppression. Neuropathy has been reported, as well as serotonin-like syndrome in patients receiving serotonergic agents. **Warning:** Lactic acidosis has been reported.

Chloramphenicol, Metronidazole

Chloramphenicol

Mode of Action

Inhibition of protein synthesis, 50s ribosome site. Bacteriostatic. Broad spectrum—gram-positive, gram-negative, *Rickettsia, Chlamydia. Pseudomonas* usually resistant. Resistance in previously sensitive organisms may occur—use sensitivity test guidance. Useful in vancomycin-resistant *E faecium* infections.

Pharmacology

Rapid oral absorption—wide distribution, including CSF; hepatic inactivation; may be used even if renal insufficiency present.

Toxicity

Fatal aplastic anemia or other dyscrasias in approximately 1 in 40,000 cases—not dose related—may occur well after cessation of therapy. Dose-related blood dyscrasias (reversible) occur more often, eg, anemia. Gray syndrome—premature and neonates—abdominal distention, vasomotor collapse, hypothermia, gray cyanosis—thus dosage to neonates should be limited to under 25 mg/kg. Other side effects—GI (disturbed resident flora), neuritis, depression (rare).

Drug	General Antibacterial Activity	Route	Usual Adult Dosage
chloramphenicol	*S typhi*, *Salmonella*, *H influenzae, Rickettsia*, *Bacteroides*, other anaerobes vancomycin-resistant *E faecium*	P.O.	50-100 mg/kg/d q 6 h*
		IV	50-100 mg/kg/d q 6 h in 4 divided doses*
metronidazole	anaerobic; gram-negative bacilli, gram-positive bacilli, and some cocci	IV	loading dose: 15 mg/kg; then
		IV	7.5 mg/kg q 6 h
		P.O.	7.5 mg/kg q 6 h
	amebiasis: liver abscess, dysentery	P.O.	500-750 mg q 8 h for 5-10 d
	Trichomonas sp	P.O.	In females: 1 g b.i.d. for 2 doses or 2 g/d as single dose

* Should not be used when other agents are available.

Indications:
1. Typhoid—resistance in Mexico and Southeast Asia;
2. Rickettsial diseases—may be superseded by equally effective tetracyclines; IV therapy if needed;
3. Melioidosis—drug of choice;
4. Tularemia—if resistant to streptomycin;
5. Plague—if resistant to streptomycin;
6. Ophthalmic infections—topical;
7. Resistant *Bacteroides;*
8. Serious infections of unknown etiology, eg, bacterial meningitis;
9. Infections where other antibiotics excluded due to state of patient, eg, renal failure meningitis in penicillin-allergic patients, meningitis due to ampicillin-resistant *Haemophilus*.

1

Metronidazole

Imidazole derivative, metabolized by the liver. Very active against gram-negative anaerobes (less active against gram-positive cocci), amebae, *Trichomonas*. Used in combination with antibiotics for polymicrobial infections. Disulfiram reactions with alcohol; potentiates anticoagulants. Agents that induce microsomal enzymes may decrease plasma metronidazole level. Carcinogenesis reported in mice and rats.

Usual Pediatric Dosage (after 3 mo of age)	Serum Binding %	Serum T½		Some Common Side Effects/Comments
		Normal	Oliguria	
50-100 mg/kg/d	25	1-2 h	3-5 h	To be reserved for serious infection—eg, *H influenzae* meningitis, typhoid fever not treated with other antimicrobials. Produces blood dyscrasias, gray syndrome. Not indicated for typhoid carriers. Seldom indicated for oral use. Rarely, has been associated with aplastic anemia.
Pediatric dosage not established, except for amebiasis	20	8 h	?	Useful in serious anaerobic infection; additional antibiotic necessary for polymicrobial infections, amebic dysentery, and abscess. Drug is used to treat *C difficile* colitis (not FDA approved); recent articles suggest decreased response with this agent. Metabolized by liver; use with caution at lower dosages in liver insufficiency. Toxicity: GI, CNS, neuropathy. Potentiates anticoagulants. **N.B. Reported to be carcinogenic in mice and rats.**

Lipopeptides, Glycopeptides

Vancomycin

Mode of Action

A glycopeptide that inhibits cell wall production, in gram-positive infections only. No cross-resistance with penicillins.

Pharmacology

Not well absorbed orally but active in gut. Use orally for antibiotic-associated pseudomembranous colitis. Prophylaxis for dental procedures in penicillin-allergic patients with prosthetic valves. Therapy for staphylococcal,

Drug	General Antibacterial Activity	Route	Usual Adult Dosage
vancomycin	staphylococci (methicillin-resistant *S aureus* and *S epidermidis*) enterococci (when sensitive) clostridia	IV P.O.	1-2 g/d 0.5-2.0 g/d
daptomycin	*S aureus*, including MRSA, GISA*, VRSA* *S pyogenes* *S pneumoniae* *S agalactiae* *S dysgalactiae* *E faecalis* (vancomycin resistant) *C jeikeium** *S hemolyticus** *S epidermidis** VRE*	IV	4 mg/kg q 24 h for complicated skin/skin structure infections. If creatinine clearance is <30 mL/min, then 4 mg/kg q 48 h. 6 mg/kg q 24h being studied for serious MSSA and MRSA infections, including bacteremia and endocarditis.

* Not FDA approved for these strains.

enterococcal infection in penicillin-cephalosporin-allergic individual. Enterococcal resistance is increasing. Resistant strains, both intermediate (GISA) and total (VRSA), have been reported.

Daptomycin

A new lipopeptide that is active and bactericidal against gram-positive organisms, daptomycin has a mode of action different from that of other antimicrobials by binding to the cell membrane, leading to the death of the organism.

Usual Pediatric Dosage (after 3 mo of age)	Serum Binding %	Serum T½		Some Common Side Effects/Comments
		Normal	Oliguria	
40 mg/kg/d IV or P.O.: 3-4 divided doses	10	6 h	240 h	Administer slowly IV. Ototoxic; nephrotoxicity increased with aminoglycosides; phlebitis. Used for methicillin-resistant *S aureus* and *S epidermidis*. Useful for staphylococcal infections in penicillin-allergic patients and for antibiotic-associated colitis (oral). Accumulates in renal failure; adjust dosage. Resistance noted in some gram-positive cocci, ie, *Leuconostoc*, *Pediococcus* and *Lactobacillus*. Resistance in enterococcal strains increasing, especially *E faecium* and some strains of *S aureus*.
not indicated	92	8.1 h	15 h	Elevated CPK may occur, as well as myopathy. Monitor at least weekly if drug is given more than 1 wk. HMG CoA reductase inhibitors (statins) should not be given.

continued on next page

Lipopeptides, Glycopeptides *(continued)*

Drug	General Antibacterial Activity	Route	Usual Adult Dosage
teicoplanin *(experimental)*	staphylococci (MRSA and *S epidermidis*), enterococci, clostridia	IV	1-2 g/d
dalbavancin*	MSSA MRSA coagulase-negative staphylococci	IV	1 g/week x 1, then 500 mg q week for skin and skin structure infections.

*Not FDA approved as of this writing.

Usual Pediatric Dosage (after 3 mo of age)	Serum Binding %	Serum $T\frac{1}{2}$		Some Common Side Effects/Comments
		Normal	Oliguria	
?	?	35-40 h	—	More potent in vitro than vancomycin; longer $T\frac{1}{2}$ should decrease dosing interval.
Not known				

Trimethoprim/ Sulfamethoxazole (TMP/SMX)

Sequential double-block of folate synthesis. Trimethoprim blocks conversion of dihydrofolate to tetrahydrofolate, while sulfonamides inhibit formation of dihydrofolate. Synergistic effect—raised activity and widened spectrum compared to sulfonamides. Formulation (80 mg TMP + 400 mg SMX) affords proper in vivo ratios in urine and blood. Pharmacokinetics of each ingredient similar. Three fatalities in otherwise healthy children, occurring over a period of 12 years, reported to the FDA; children developed Stevens-Johnson syndrome while being treated with TMP/SMX.

Has very broad in vitro spectrum, including bacteria, *Chlamydia*, *Nocardia*,

Drug	Indications*	Route
trimethoprim/ sulfamethoxazole (TMP/SMX)	*Shigella* severe urinary tract infections due to susceptible strains *Pneumocystis jiroveci* pneumonitis (use for other serious infections is pending) methicillin-resistant *S aureus* (MRSA) infections have been treated successfully (drug not approved for this organism)	IV ↓

*Some indications not approved.

Trimethoprim

A synthetic antibacterial agent that blocks production of tetrahydrofolic acid from dihydrofolic acid by inhibiting dihydrofolate reductase. For use in urinary tract infections caused by *E coli*, *Klebsiella*, *Proteus mirabilis*, and *Enterobacter* sp. Toxicities are the same as those associated with the sulfonamides.

Drug	Serum $T\frac{1}{2}$		Approximate Urine Solubility	Usual Adult Dosage
	Normal	Oliguria		
trimethoprim	8-10 h		+++	100 mg b.i.d. for 10 d or 200 mg q.d. x 10 d

\+ = less
+++ = more

Pneumocystis carinii, Rickettsia, Legionella. Available in IV preparation.

Indications

1. Urinary tract infection: Active vs *E coli, Klebsiella, Enterobacter, Proteus mirabilis, Proteus* (indole positive), *Serratia*; useful in prostatitis;
2. Other infections: Shigellosis, otitis media due to ampicillin-resistant *Haemophilus* and *S pneumoniae*, lung infection, lymphogranuloma, salmonellosis, *Brucella, P jiroveci, N gonorrhoeae.*

Toxicity

Same as for sulfonamides. Folate deficiency rare with prolonged therapy. Trimethoprim may be toxic to neonate and fetus. Avoid in lactating women.

Dosage (Adults and Children)	Serum Binding %	Serum T½		Common Side Effects/ Comments
		Normal	Oliguria	
(based on trimethoprim) 8-10 mg/kg/d, in divided doses, q 6-12 h for 14 d	trimethoprim: 44	11 h	decreased	Not effective against *Pseudomonas.* Use ½ normal dose when creatinine clearance is 15-30 mL/min.
15-20 mg/kg/d, in divided doses, trimethoprim q 6-8 h for 14-21 d	sulfamethoxazole: 70	12 h		Diffuses well into CSF. Useful in prophylaxis of *P carinii* pneumonia.

Usual Pediatric Dosage	Usual Dose Frequency (doses/d)	Some Common Side Effects/Comments
not established	2	Resistance has been reported. Used as prophylaxis in urinary tract infections. Same side effects as those of sulfonamides.

The Sulfonamides

Mode of Action and Pharmacology

Bacteriostatic—interfere with folic acid synthesis by competition with para-aminobenzoic acid (PABA). Sensitivity tests unreliable. Diffuse well after absorption. Most used in urinary infection and *Nocardia* infection.

Classification of Sulfonamides

1. Short-acting (half-life 4-7 h): Considered preparations of choice. Give every 4-8 h. Little difference between types.
2. Medium long-acting (half-life 10-12 h): Absorbed and excreted more slowly. Give once or twice daily. Useful for longer therapy.
3. Long-acting (half-life 17-40 h): Very slow excretion. Once-daily administration.
4. Ultra long-acting (half-life 65-200 h): Not available in United States.
5. Unabsorbed sulfonamides: Used for colonic sterilization.
6. Topical sulfonamides: Burns (mafenide, silver sulfadiazine). Eye infections: sulfacetamide. Other topical use not recommended (contact dermatitis, resistance).
7. Combination with trimethoprim: See section on trimethoprim/sulfamethoxazole (TMP/SMX).

Side Effects and Toxicology

GI: Nausea, vomiting, abdominal pain, diarrhea (rare).
Renal: Crystalluria, hematuria (inadequate flow and alkalinization), use with great care in renal failure. Hypersensitivity rare.

Drug	Serum $T^1/_2$ Normal	Serum $T^1/_2$ Oliguria	Approximate Urine Solubility	Usual Adult Dosage
A. Short-acting				
sulfisoxazole	5-7 h	12 h	+++	P.O.: 0.5-1 g q 6 h IV: 4-8 g/d in 4-6 divided doses
sulfadiazine	2-5 h	12-25 h	+	2-4 g/d in 3-6 divided doses
B. Medium long-acting				
sulfa-methoxazole	9 h	25 h	+++	2 g/d in 2 divided doses

+ = less
+++ = more

Hematologic: Hemolytic anemia (G6PD deficiency), methemoglobinemia, hemoglobinuria, granulocytopenia, aplastic anemia, pancytopenia, etc, bone marrow toxicity.
Dermatologic: Rashes, photosensitivity, contact dermatitis.
Hypersensitivity: Stevens-Johnson syndrome, exfoliative dermatitis, epidermal necrolysis, erythema multiforme, erythema nodosum, Behçet's syndrome. Fever, arthralgia, serum sickness, anaphylaxis (rare). Pulmonary eosinophilia.
Other side effects: Goiter, drug interactions (sulfonylureas, coumarin), porphyria exacerbation, neonatal hyperbilirubinemia. Occasional neurologic side effects. Interference with laboratory urine tests—false-positive Benedict's, albumin, urobilinogen, porphyrins.

Precautions in Use

1. Unreliable sensitivity tests—clinical judgment needed.
2. Maintain urine output (1.2 L/d). Alkalinize if using sulfadiazine and sulfamethoxazole.
3. Do not use longer-acting types.
4. If hypersensitive to one sulfonamide, avoid all sulfonamides.
5. Do not use during third trimester, for neonates, or for premature infants.
6. Patient instructions should include: look for rash, fever, jaundice, purpura.

Indications

Lower Urinary Tract Infections: Especially *E coli, P mirabilis, Klebsiella*; TMP/SMX more effective. Nocardiosis, some protozoal infections. Prophylaxis for rheumatic fever in penicillin-allergic patient. *Note:* not for treatment of group A streptococcus infection.

Usual Pediatric Dosage (after 3 mo of age)	Usual Dose Frequency (doses/d)	Some Common Side Effects/ Comments
loading dose ½ regular dose; then 100-150 mg/kg/d in 4-6 divided doses	4-6	Alkalinization of urine allows more solubility. Contraindicated in pregnancy, at term, or during the nursing period.
100-150 mg/kg/d in 4-6 divided doses	4-6	Systemic use, less satisfactory for urinary infections.
50-60 mg/kg/d in 2 divided doses	2	Maintain high fluid, perhaps alkalinize.

Urinary Antibacterials

Nitrofurantoin: Nitrofurans toxic, but nitrofurantoin quickly excreted in urine so toxic blood levels not reached. Broad-spectrum, especially gram-negative—*E coli*, *Klebsiella*, *Enterobacter*, *Proteus* (indole positive), enterococci. Most *Proteus* and *Pseudomonas* not inhibited. Toxicity and side effects more common than with sulfonamides, especially GI. Should not be used in patients in renal failure. Macrocrystalline form may be more tolerable. Can produce fever, rash, eosinophilia, and pulmonary infiltrates.

Trimethoprim/Sulfamethoxazole TMP/SMX: See section on page 78 about this combination agent.

Nalidixic Acid: Inhibits DNA synthesis. Wide gram-negative spectrum. Resistance to nalidixic acid commonly occurs during treatment. Not to be

Drug	General Antibacterial Activity	Route	Usual Adult Dosage
nitrofurantoin	*E coli* enterococci *S aureus* *Klebsiella* *Aerobacter*	P.O.	50-100 mg q 6 h
trimethoprim + sulfamethoxazole (TMP/SMX)	*E coli* *Klebsiella* *Enterobacter* *Proteus* *Serratia*	P.O. IV	80-160 mg TMP + 400-800 mg SMX, b.i.d. based on 3-5 mg/kg/d of TMP* in 2-4 divided doses
nalidixic acid	gram-negatives, except *Pseudomonas*	P.O.	1 g q 6 h
cinoxacin	gram-negatives, except *Pseudomonas*	P.O.	250-500 mg q 6 h
methenamine	Action due to liberation of formaldehyde. Most organisms sensitive.	P.O.	
methenamine mandelate methenamine hippurate	Maintain urine acidity—otherwise use acidulants.		mandelate—1 g after each meal and at bedtime hippurate—1 g b.i.d.

* Higher dosage necessary for treatment of *Pneumocystis jiroveci* pneumonia.

used in patients with renal insufficiency. Side effects not common in short-term use. Gastrointestinal, photosensitivity, and neurologic. Not indicated in neonates and infants. Resistance may develop rapidly.

Methenamine: Hydrolyzed in acid urine to formaldehyde. Most urinary pathogens susceptible, but *Pseudomonas*, *Proteus*, *Enterobacter* most resistant. Used for long-term suppression—fewer side effects than sulfonamides. Patient must be able to acidify urine—commercial preparations use mandelic or hippuric acids. Can use cranberry juice (hippuric acid), ascorbic acid, or ammonium chloride.

Cinoxacin: Similar to nalidixic acid; less GI intolerance.

Poorly Absorbed Antibiotics

Indanyl carbenicillin: See 'Penicillins.'

Usual Pediatric Dose (after 3 mo of age)	Some Common Side Effects/Comments
5-7 mg/kg/d divided q 6 h	*Proteus* and *Pseudomonas* resistant. GI, hypersensitivity—rashes, fever, pulmonary infiltrates, and fibrosis. Neurologic—peripheral neuropathy, cerebral symptoms. Hematologic—marrow depression, hemolytic anemia (G6PD deficiency)—jaundice rare. Do not use in infants under 1 month old.
6-12 mg/kg/d (based on TMP) in 2-4 divided doses	As for sulfonamides. Long-term folate deficiency. Contraindicated in last trimester, lactation, neonate, megaloblastic anemia. Caution in renal and liver disease. Trimethoprim serum half-life (h)—normal: 10; oliguria: 25. Sulfamethoxazole serum half-life (h)—normal: 9; oliguria: 25. Penetrates CNS.
55 mg/kg/d divided q 6 h	GI, photosensitivity, fever, eosinophilia, neurologic disorders, visual disturbances. Mild hematologic disorders. Use full dose to limit emergence of resistance. Avoid with renal insufficiency.
not recommended	Less GI distress than with nalidixic acid.
age 6-12 yr: ½ adult dose	Use only for long-term therapy—as urinary antiseptic not tissue infection, eg, pyelonephritis. Maintain acid urine. Few side effects—GI, rash, dysuria.

The Fluoroquinolones

The fluoroquinolones (commonly known as quinolones) are a class of synthetic antibacterial agents that possess a broad spectrum of antimicrobial activity. Many of the fluoroquinolones have varying degrees of in vitro activity against *Chlamydia*, *Mycoplasma*, *Mycobacterium*, *Ureaplasma*, and *Legionella*.

This class possesses excellent pharmacokinetic properties; they are

Drug	General Antibacterial Activity*	Route	Usual Adult Dosage
cipro-floxacin	*P aeruginosa* *Serratia* *Enterobacter* sp Enterobacteriaceae eg, *E coli* *Klebsiella* sp *Shigella* sp *Salmonella* sp *Campylobacter* sp *N gonorrhoeae* *H influenzae* Some *S aureus* (MSSA only) less active *S pneumoniae*	P.O. oral suspension	intra-abdominal: complicated: 500 mg q 12 h x 7 to 14 d (used in conjunction with metronidazole) bone and joint: mild/moderate: 500 mg q 12 h ≥4 to 6 wk severe/complicated: 750 mg q 12 h ≥4 to 6 wk infectious diarrhea: mild/moderate/severe: 500 mg q 12 h x 5 to 7 d urethral and cervical gonococcal infections: uncomplicated: 250 mg single dose chronic bacterial prostatitis: mild/moderate: 500 mg q 12 h x 28 d acute uncomplicated (*E coli*) pyelonephritis: XR 1,000 mg x 7-14 d** sinusitis, mild/moderate: acute: 500 mg q 12 h x 10 d lower respiratory tract; skin and skin structure: mild/moderate: 500 mg q 12 h x 7 to 14 d severe/complicated: 750 mg q 12 h x 7 to 14 d typhoid fever: mild/moderate: 500 mg q 12 h x 10 d urinary tract: acute uncomplicated: 250 mg b.i.d. x 3 d or XR 500 mg x 3 d** mild/moderate: 250 mg q 12 h x 7 to 14 d severe/complicated: 500 mg q 12 h x 7 to 14 d or XR 1,000 mg x 7-14 d**
		IV only	nosocomial pneumonia: mild/moderate/severe: 400 mg q 12 h

*Treatment of gram-negative bacteremia in granulocytopenic hosts probably should be with two agents to which bacteria are sensitive and/or synergistic. Gram-negative pneumonia probably requires two agents.

**Do not crush, split, or chew tablet.

absorbed orally, with good bioavailability and wide tissue distribution. Many have an extended $T^1/_2$ (half-life), allowing for once- or twice-daily dosing and enhancement of patient compliance. Some agents are metabolized, while others are excreted unchanged.

Other favorable properties include lack of cross-allergenicity to the β-lactams and favorable side effect profiles.

Levofloxacin, moxifloxacin, gatifloxacin, and gemifloxacin possess the

Usual Pediatric Dosage	Serum Binding %	Serum $T^1/_2$ Normal	Serum $T^1/_2$ Oliguria	Common Side Effects/ Comments
not indicated	20-40	4-5 h	4-7 h	Aluminum- and magnesium-based antacids decrease absorption. GI side effects: nausea 5.2%, diarrhea 2.3%. CNS side effects: restlessness, insomnia are increased in elderly; theophylline, caffeine and warfarin metabolism may be decreased and serum levels may increase. Rarely, seizures reported. May interact with NSAIDs.* *Warnings:* Should not be used in children or pregnant women. The QTc interval may be prolonged, so caution must be used in patients on drugs that increase QTc and for medical conditions that are associated with increased QTc.

* NSAID = nonsteroidal anti-inflammatory drug

continued on next page

highest gram-positive activity, while ciprofloxacin is still the most active antipseudomonal agent.

Quinolones have found increasing clinical utility because of their spectrum and their excellent pharmacokinetics. All are well absorbed after oral administration and most have tissue concentrations in excess of serum levels, although half-lives tend to vary. Some are given b.i.d. or, more recently, q.d., enhancing patient compliance. Some agents require dosage

Drug	General Antibacterial Activity*	Route	Usual Adult Dosage
ciprofloxacin *(continued)*	*P aeruginosa* *Serratia* *Enterobacter* sp Enterobacteriaceae eg, *E coli* *Klebsiella* sp *Shigella* sp *Salmonella* sp *Campylobacter* sp *N gonorrhoeae* *H influenzae* Some *S aureus* (MSSA only) less active *S pneumoniae*	IV	intra-abdominal: complicated: 400 mg IV q 12 h or 500 mg P.O. q 12 h (used in conjunction with metronidazole) febrile neutropenia, severe: 400 mg IV q 8 h + 50 mg/kg q 4 h, plus piperacillin/tazobactam lower respiratory tract: mild to moderate: 400 mg IV q 2 h or 500 mg P.O. q 12 h severe: 400 mg IV q 8 h or 750 mg P.O. q 12 h skin/skin structure and bone/joint: mild to moderate: 400 mg IV q 12 h or 500 mg P.O. q 12 h severe: 400 mg IV q 8 h or 750 mg P.O. q 12 h urinary tract: mild to moderate: 200 mg IV q 12 h or 250 mg P.O. q 12 h severe: 400 mg IV q 12 h or 500 mg P.O. q 12 h
	Bacillus anthracis (anthrax)	IV	Treatment: 400 mg IV q 12 h x 60 d
		P.O.	Prophylaxis: 500 mg q 12 h x 60 d
		otic	acute otitis externa: for adults and children 1 year old and older, 3 drops into ear b.i.d. x 7 d

*Treatment of gram-negative bacteremia in granulocytopenic hosts probably should be with two agents to which bacteria are sensitive and/or synergistic. Gram-negative pneumonia probably requires two agents.

adjustment in renally impaired patients, while others, such as moxifloxacin, have a balanced elimination, thereby not leading to accumulation in cases of organ dysfunction. Metabolism also plays a major role in drug-drug interactions. Those quinolones that are metabolized via the cytochrome P-450 pathway will interact with or inhibit other drugs that are also metabolized through this route. Moxifloxacin and levofloxacin have no interaction with theophylline and caffeine.

All quinolones are negatively affected by multivalent cations (Al^{+++},

Usual Pediatric Dosage	Serum Binding %	Serum T½ Normal	Serum T½ Oliguria	Common Side Effects/ Comments
indicated for children 1 year old and older				

continued on next page

Mg^{++}, Fe^{++}, etc) so that absorption is significantly decreased. Therefore, staggered dosing is recommended to avoid underdosing.

Quinolones have been investigated in a wide range of infections, including pulmonary, urinary, skin and soft-tissue, osteomyelitis, intra-abdominal, gastrointestinal, STDs, and septicemia. Because of their broadening spectrum of activity, some with activity against multiresistant *S pneumoniae*, the newer quinolones are being considered as a significant option in community-acquired respiratory infections. Moxifloxacin, levofloxacin, gatifloxacin, and gemifloxacin are being investigated in DRSP infections. Although these new agents have better gram-positive activity, they should not be used in MRSA or VRE infections, since quinolone resistance may emerge.

Recent studies have begun to demonstrate differences between new members of the class in terms of their activity and their ability to select for resistance. Structural differences

Drug	General Antibacterial Activity*	Route	Usual Adult Dosage
gatifloxacin	*S aureus* (methicillin-susceptible strains) *S pneumoniae* (penicillin-susceptible strains) *E coli* *H influenzae* *H parainfluenzae* *K influenzae* *K parainfluenzae* *M catarrhalis* *N gonorrhoeae* *P mirabilis* *C pneumoniae* *L pneumophila* *M pneumoniae*	P.O. IV	acute bacterial exacerbations of chronic bronchitis: 400 mg q 24 h x 5 d cystitis: 200 mg q 24 h x 3 d or 400 mg x 1 dose uncomplicated gonorrhea: 400 mg single dose community-acquired pneumonia: 400 mg q 24 h x 7-14 d pyelonephritis: 400 mg q 24 h x 7-10 d acute maxillary sinusitis: 400 mg q 24 h x 10 d complicated UTI: 400 mg q 24 h x 7-10 d

*Treatment of gram-negative bacteremia in granulocytopenic hosts probably should be with two agents to which bacteria are sensitive and/or synergistic. Gram-negative pneumonia probably requires two agents.

between quinolones at one or two positions yield varying affinities for the key targets of DA gyrase II or topoisomerase IV or the ability to withstand efflux from the cell. These mechanisms are most pronounced when the concentrations for the drug stay in the optimal range for the entire dosing period. The minimum inhibitory concentration appears to be different, based on specific structures. The possession of a methoxy group at C-8 (moxifloxacin and gatifloxacin) plays a partial role in this phenomenon.

The use of optimal dosing of the newer quinolones should help minimize the emergence of resistance, but suboptimal dosing of any quinolone could undermine what has become a valuable group of evolving antimicrobials.

The quinolones are potent oral agents that permit sequential therapy from parenteral dosing; this leads to marked savings from lower drug costs (overall), usually earlier discharge from hospital, and improvement of a patient's quality of life. Finally, the IV-PO administration has been especially welcome in the nursing home setting.

Usual Pediatric Dosage	**Serum Binding %**	**Serum $T^{1/2}$**		**Common Side Effects/ Comments**
		Normal	**Oliguria**	
not indicated	20	7-8 h	prolonged	Aluminum- and magnesium-based antacids decrease absorption. No interactions with cyclosporine, theophylline, or warfarin. Hyperglycemia and hypoglycemia have been reported, usually in diabetics on oral hypoglycemics or insulin. The elderly, patients with renal failure, and other medical conditions may be at increased risk. Elevated digoxin levels have been reported in volunteer studies.* Dosage adjustment necessary for renal insufficiency. *Warnings:* Should not be used in children or pregnant women. The QTc interval may be prolonged, so caution must be used in patients on drugs that increase QTc and for medical conditions that are associated with increased QTc.

* See package insert

continued on next page

The Fluoroquinolones *(continued)*

Drug	General Antibacterial Activity*	Route	Usual Adult Dosage
gemifloxacin	*E coli* *Enterobacter* *Serratia* sp *Campylobacter* sp *P aeruginosa* *N gonorrhoeae* *M catarrhalis* *H influenzae* *S aureus* *S pneumoniae*** *C trachomatis* Some MRSA *K pneumoniae* *M pneumoniae* *M catarrhalis* *C pneumoniae* *L pneumoniae* *Salmonella* sp *Shigella* sp Effective against multidrug-resistant *S pneumoniae*	P.O.	AECB: 320 mg P.O. q.d. x 5 d community-acquired pneumonia: 320 mg P.O. q.d. x 7 d

*Treatment of gram-negative bacteremia in granulocytopenic hosts probably should be with two agents to which bacteria are sensitive and/or synergistic. Gram-negative pneumonia probably requires two agents.

**Including penicillin-resistant *S pneumoniae.*

1

Usual Pediatric Dosage	Serum Binding %	Serum $T_{1/2}$ Normal	Serum $T_{1/2}$ Oliguria	Common Side Effects/ Comments
not indicated	60-70	7 h	increased	Aluminum- and magnesium-based antacids decrease absorption; dizziness may occur. Nausea: 3%. May interact with NSAIDs.* Plasma levels almost equal after same IV and P.O. dose. Effective against atypical respiratory pathogens. Increased incidence in rash, especially in younger women, most often seen after 7 d of therapy. *Warnings:* Should not be used in children or pregnant women. The QTc interval may be prolonged, so caution must be used in patients on drugs that increase QTc and for medical conditions that are associated with increased QTc.

* NSAID = nonsteroidal anti-inflammatory drug

continued on next page

The Fluoroquinolones *(continued)*

Drug	General Antibacterial Activity	Route	Usual Adult Dosage
levofloxacin	*E coli* *Enterobacter* *Serratia* sp *Campylobacter* sp *P aeruginosa* *N gonorrhoeae* *M catarrhalis* *H influenzae* *S aureus* *S pneumoniae** *C trachomatis* Some MRSA *K pneumoniae* *M pneumoniae* *M catarrhalis* *C pneumoniae* *L pneumoniae* *Salmonella* sp *Shigella* sp	P.O. IV	acute bacterial exacerbations of chronic bronchitis: 500 mg q 24 h x 7 d community-acquired pneumonia (mild to moderate): 750 mg q.d. x 5 d nosocomial pneumonia: 750 mg q.d. x 7-14 d acute pyelonephritis: 250 mg q 24 h x 10 d acute bacterial sinusitis: 750 mg q 24 h x 5 d uncomplicated skin/skin structure: 500 mg q 24 h x 7-10 d complicated UTI: 250 mg q 24 h x 10 d
lomefloxacin	*S saprophyticus* *E coli* *C diversus* *E cloacae* *H influenzae* *M catarrhalis* *P mirabilis* *P aeruginosa* (urinary tract only)	P.O.	lower respiratory tract infections**: 400 mg/d x 10 d for prophylaxis of transurethral surgical procedures: 400 mg 2-6 h before surgery urinary tract: cystitis: 400 mg/d x 10 d complicated urinary tract infections: 400 mg/d x 14 d

* Including penicillin-resistant *S pneumoniae*.

** Only for acute bacterial exacerbations of chronic bronchitis caused by *M catarrhalis* or *H influenzae*, not *S pneumoniae*.

Usual Pediatric Dosage	Serum Binding %	Serum $T^{1}/_{2}$ Normal	Serum $T^{1}/_{2}$ Oliguria	Common Side Effects/ Comments
not indicated	24-38	6-8 h	pro-longed	Aluminum- and magnesium-based antacids decrease absorption; dizziness may occur. Nausea: 3%. May interact with NSAIDs.* *Warnings:* Should not be used in children or pregnant women. Plasma levels almost equal after same IV and P.O. dose. Effective against atypical respiratory pathogens. The QTc interval may be prolonged, so caution must be used in patients on drugs that increase QTc and for medical conditions that are associated with increased QTc.
not indicated	10	7.75 h	21 h	Aluminum- and magnesium-based antacids decrease absorption; dizziness may occur. Nausea: 3%. May interact with NSAIDs.* Less interaction with theophylline than other quinolones. *Warnings:* Should not be used in children or pregnant women. The QTc interval may be prolonged, so caution must be used in patients on drugs that increase QTc and for medical conditions that are associated with increased QTc.

* NSAID = nonsteroidal anti-inflammatory drug

continued on next page

The Fluoroquinolones *(continued)*

Drug	General Antibacterial Activity*	Route	Usual Adult Dosage
moxifloxacin	*S pneumoniae* *H influenzae* (including beta-lactamase+)	P.O. IV	acute exacerbation of chronic bronchitis: 400 mg q.d. x 5 d
	M catarrhalis (including beta-lactamase+) *H parainfluenzae*	P.O.	community-acquired pneumonia (mild to moderate) 400 mg q.d. x 10 d
	S aureus *S pyogenes* *K pneumoniae*	IV	community-acquired pneumonia: 400 mg q.d. x 7-14 d
	C pneumoniae *M pneumoniae* *S pneumoniae***	P.O. IV	acute sinusitis: 400 mg q.d. x 10 d
	(penicillin-resistant) *L pneumophila*** *Fusobacterium* sp** *Peptostreptococcus* sp** *Prevotella* sp** *P mirabilis*** *M tuberculosis***	IV	uncomplicated skin/skin structure infections: 400 mg q.d. x 7 d
norfloxacin	staphylococci, *E faecalis*, gram-negative bacilli	P.O.	urinary tract infections complicated UTI: 400 mg b.i.d. x 10-21 d for elderly or those with renal impairment, adjust dosage (see package insert) uncomplicated: 400 mg b.i.d. x 7-10 d

*Treatment of gram-negative bacteremia in granulocytopenic hosts probably should be with two agents to which bacteria are sensitive and/or synergistic. Gram-negative pneumonia probably requires two agents.

**In vitro susceptibility only.

1

Usual Pediatric Dosage	Serum Binding %	Serum $T_{1/2}$		Common Side Effects/ Comments
		Normal	Oliguria	
not indicated	45	12 h	12 h	Interactions with aluminum- and magnesium-containing antacids, sucralfate, and iron. No interactions with theophylline, ranitidine, morphine, warfarin, calcium, oral contraceptives, digoxin, caffeine, glyburide, dairy products, or food. No need to adjust dosing in renal dysfunction or mild-to-moderate hepatic dysfunction. No dosage adjustment when switching from IV to P.O. Avoid concomitant medications known to prolong QTc. *Warnings:* Should not be used in children or pregnant women. The QTc interval may be prolonged, so caution must be used in patients on drugs that increase QTc and for medical conditions that are associated with increased QTc.
not indicated	15-30	1.7 h	3-4 h	Take with one glass of water 1 h before or 2 h after a meal. Avoid concomitant antacids, or within 2 h of dosing. Caution in elderly patients; side effects include crystalluria and dizziness or lightheadedness. *Warnings:* Should not be used in children or pregnant women. The QTc interval may be prolonged, so caution must be used in patients on drugs that increase QTc and for medical conditions that are associated with increased QTc.

continued on next page

The Fluoroquinolones *(continued)*

Drug	General Antibacterial Activity*	Route	Usual Adult Dosage
ofloxacin	*Enterobacter* *Serratia* sp *Salmonella* sp *Shigella* sp *Campylobacter* sp *P aeruginosa* *N gonorrhoeae* *M catarrhalis* *H influenzae* *S aureus* *S pneumoniae* *C trachomatis*	P.O. IV(1) (1) See package insert for full prescribing information	urinary tract cystitis due to *E coli*, *K pneumoniae*: 200 mg b.i.d. x 3 d, or 200 mg b.i.d. x 7 d if due to other organisms prostatitis due to *E coli*.** 300 mg b.i.d. x 6 wk lower respiratory tract: 400 mg b.i.d. x 10 d Sexually transmitted disease *C trachomatis*, with or without *N gonorrhoeae*: 300 mg b.i.d. x 7 d *N gonorrhoeae*, acute, uncomplicated: 400 mg x 1 dose skin/skin structure mild to moderate: 400 mg b.i.d. x 10 d complicated UTI: 200 mg b.i.d. x 10 d

*Treatment of gram-negative bacteremia in granulocytopenic hosts probably should be with two agents to which bacteria are sensitive and/or synergistic. Gram-negative pneumonia probably requires two agents.

**Because there are no safety data presently available to support the use of IV ofloxacin for more than 10 days, therapy thereafter should be switched to oral tablet or to other appropriate therapy.

Usual Pediatric Dosage	Serum Binding %	Serum T½ Normal	Serum T½ Oliguria	Common Side Effects/ Comments
not indicated	32	6 h	9-25 h	Aluminum- and magnesium-based antacids decrease absorption; dizziness may occur. Nausea: 3%. May interact with NSAIDs.* Caution with use of theophylline and warfarin. *Warnings:* Should not be used in children or pregnant women. The QTc interval may be prolonged, so caution must be used in patients on drugs that increase QTc and for medical conditions that are associated with increased QTc.

*NSAID = nonsteroidal anti-inflammatory drug

continued on next page

The Fluoroquinolones *(continued)*

Drug	General Antibacterial Activity	Route	Usual Adult Dosage
trova-floxacin **should not be used if safer therapy avail-able†**	*S aureus* (methicillin-sensitive only) *S agalactiae* *S pneumoniae* (penicillin-susceptible and penicillin-resistant*) *S pyogenes* *Viridans* group streptococci *E coli* *G vaginalis* *H influenzae* *K pneumoniae* *M catarrhalis* *P aeruginosa*** *P vulgaris** *B fragilis* *Peptostreptococcus* sp *Prevotella* sp *C pneumoniae* *L pneumophila* *M pneumoniae* *E faecalis****	P.O. or IV	**Used only in serious or life-threatening infections:** complicated intra-abdominal infections including postsurgical infections: 300 mg IV followed by 200 mg P.O. q.d. x 7-14 d gynecologic and pelvic infections: 300 mg IV followed by 200 mg P.O. q.d. x 7-14 d community-acquired pneumonia: 200 mg P.O. or 200 mg IV followed by 200 mg P.O. q.d. x 7-14 d nosocomial pneumonia: 300 mg IV followed by 200 mg P.O. q.d. x 10-14 d complicated skin and skin structure infections including diabetic foot infections: 200 mg P.O. or 200 mg IV followed by 200 mg P.O. q.d. 10-14 d

* Active in vitro but clinical significance unknown.

** Use of aztreonam or an aminoglycoside may be indicated.

*** Used in mixed skin infections.

† **Trovafloxacin should not be used when safer, alternative antimicrobial therapy may be effective.** Trovafloxacin has been associated with serious liver injury leading to liver transplantation and/or death. Trovafloxacin-associated liver injury has been reported with both short-term and long-term drug exposure.

Usual Pediatric Dosage	Serum Binding %	Serum $T^{1/2}$		Common Side Effects/ Comments
		Normal	Oliguria	
not indicated for patients <18 years of age	76%	9-13 h	9-13h	Aluminum- and magnesium-containing antacids, sucralfate, ferrous sulfate, intravenous morphine, calcium carbonate, and omeprazole all decrease absorption. Increases caffeine exposure. Most common side effects include dizziness, nausea, headache, and lightheadedness. No dosage adjustments needed in patients with renal failure. *Warnings:* Should not be used in children or pregnant women. The QTc interval may be prolonged, so caution must be used in patients on drugs that increase QTc and for medical conditions that are associated with increased QTc.

continued on next page

The Fluoroquinolones *(continued)*

Drug	General Antibacterial Activity	Route	Usual Adult Dosage
trova-floxacin **should not be used if safer therapy available**†	*S aureus* (methicillin-sensitive only) *S agalactiae* *S pneumoniae* (penicillin-susceptible and penicillin-resistant*) *S pyogenes* *Viridans* group streptococci *E coli* *G vaginalis* *H influenzae* *K pneumoniae* *M catarrhalis* *P aeruginosa*** *P vulgaris** *B fragilis* *Peptostreptococcus* sp *Prevotella* sp *C pneumoniae* *L pneumophila* *M pneumoniae* *E faecalis****	P.O. or IV	**Used only in serious or life-threatening infections:** complicated intra-abdominal infections including postsurgical infections: 300 mg IV followed by 200 mg P.O. q.d. x 7-14 d gynecologic and pelvic infections: 300 mg IV followed by 200 mg P.O. q.d. x 7-14 d community-acquired pneumonia: 200 mg P.O. or 200 mg IV followed by 200 mg P.O. q.d. x 7-14 d nosocomial pneumonia: 300 mg IV followed by 200 mg P.O. q.d. x 10-14 d complicated skin and skin structure infections including diabetic foot infections: 200 mg P.O. or 200 mg IV followed by 200 mg P.O. q.d. 10-14 d

* Active in vitro but clinical significance unknown.
** Use of aztreonam or an aminoglycoside may be indicated.
*** Used in mixed skin infections.
† **Trovafloxacin should not be used when safer, alternative antimicrobial therapy may be effective.** Trovafloxacin has been associated with serious liver injury leading to liver transplantation and/or death. Trovafloxacin-associated liver injury has been reported with both short-term and long-term drug exposure.

Usual Pediatric Dosage	Serum Binding %	Serum T½		Common Side Effects/ Comments
		Normal	Oliguria	
				Trovafloxacin-associated liver enzyme abnormalities, symptomatic hepatitis, jaundice, and liver failure (including rare reports of acute hepatic necrosis with eosinophilic infiltration, liver transplantation and/or death) have been reported with both short-term and long-term drug exposure in men and women. Trovafloxacin use exceeding 2 wk is associated with a significantly increased risk of serious liver injury. Liver injury has also been reported following trovafloxacin re-exposure. Clinicians should monitor liver function tests (eg, AST, ALT, bilirubin) in trovafloxacin recipients who develop signs or symptoms consistent with hepatitis. Clinicians should consider discontinuing trovafloxacin in those patients who develop liver function test abnormalities. Dosage adjustments in patients with mild to moderate cirrhosis.

Tuberculosis*

Antonio Anzueto, MD

Multidrug-resistant tuberculosis (MDR-TB) cases have been increasing. If you suspect MDR-TB, a current recommendation is this regimen:

• Isoniazid (INH)	300 mg/d
• Rifampin	600 mg/d
• Pyrazinamide (PZA)	15-30 mg/kg/d maximum 2 g/d
• Ethambutol	15-25 mg/kg/d
• Pyridoxine	25 mg/d x 6 mo

All isolates should be sent for antibiotic sensitivities. This regimen is given for 2 months. If the review shows that isolates are sensitive, INH and rifampin are continued for an additional 4 months, with INH at a dose of 15 mg/kg (maximum 900 mg) and rifampin 600 mg, each given twice weekly. Otherwise, the drug regimen must be adjusted to sensitivities and those agents that are resistant are deleted and others added so that at least two active agents are given for at least 9 months.

In some urban areas, it is recommended that all new cases of tuberculosis be treated with the four-drug regimen because the incidence of MDR-TB is more than 30% in these locales. Some physicians add a quinolone to this therapy.

See treatment algorithms, Figures 1 and 2.

Isoniazid (INH): Potent. Wide distribution, including CSF—urinary excretion. Inhibits pyridoxine metabolism—neurotoxicity, convulsions, neuritis. Can add pyridoxine to regimen. Hepatotoxicity and fulminant hepatic failure have been reported. Patients should be monitored by physician periodically as well as monthly or when symptoms and signs of liver disease occur; uncommon under age 25.

Ethambutol: Well tolerated, effective. Visual disturbance, retrobulbar neuritis at higher doses. Delays onset of TB resistance with other anti-TB agents.

Quinolones: Some of these agents have been added to regimens as part of a multidrug regimen for MDR-TB.

Streptomycin: See 'Aminoglycosides.' Must be used with another agent due to rapid resistance if used alone.

***p*-aminosalicylic acid (PAS):** Delays resistance—increases INH blood levels when combined with latter. GI disturbances frequent—hepatitis, rash.

Rifampin: Potent. Excreted mainly through bile. Flulike syndrome with intermittent usage. Rare nephrotoxicity. Also used for meningococcal carriers in U.S. Also inhibits many gram-positive and gram-negative bacteria. May increase metabolism of concomitantly administered drugs.

New formulations: Rifabutin should be considered in patients receiving antiretroviral drugs. Rifapentine is given with isoniazid in a once-a-week continuation phase regimen. New formulations of rifampin compounds are available, offering better safety profiles and once-a-day dosing regimen. Fixed-dose combination preparations may minimize therapy noncompliance and decrease the frequency of acquired drug resistance.

Capreomycin: For treatment of TB in adults and adolescents, 1 g injected into the muscle once a day for 60 to 120 days. Then, 1 g injected 2 or 3 times a

*See: Initial therapy for tuberculosis in the era of multidrug resistance. *MMWR* 1993;42(RR-7):1-8, and American Thoracic Society/Centers for Disease Control and Prevention/Infectious Disease Society of America: Treatment of tuberculosis. *Am J Respir Crit Care Med* 2003;167:602-662. All strains should be tested for resistance, which has been reported to be increasing rapidly. Treatment of tuberculosis in HIV-positive patients at this time requires four drugs.

week. This agent must be given with other medicines to treat TB. Dosage for children has not been determined.
Ethionamide: May be hepatotoxic.
Pyrazinamide: Useful in combined therapy of INH-resistant strains. Hepatic toxicity. Resistance emerges after short-term therapy—should never be used alone. May produce gout.
Cycloserine: Not as effective as streptomycin or INH. Neurotoxicity, cerebral symptoms common.
Kanamycin: See 'Aminoglycosides.' More renal toxicity than streptomycin.
Clofazimine: An antileprosy agent. It has been used with other drugs to treat *Mycobacterium avium intracellulare* in AIDS patients (not released for this indication).

Nontuberculous Mycobacteria
Nontuberculous mycobacteria (atypical mycobacteria) have been associated with a variety of systemic infections. Though often isolated from the lung, bone marrow, and urine, the exact role of the organism in disease is defined by the clinical status; many isolates are probably colonizers. Definite syndromes have been noted, including pulmonary disease, lymphadenitis, soft-tissue infection with sinus formation, osteomyelitis (including sternal osteomyelitis), genitourinary infections, meningitis, eye infections, and heterograft infection. Infection occurs in immunocompromised hosts and in cases of AIDS. Different schemata for the microbiologic classification of these mycobacteria have been described, based on pigment formation or lack of it, as well as on the rapidity of growth in culture. Antibiotic treatment is difficult at best and often requires the simultaneous administration of three to five agents; cures from this regimen have been limited and surgical extirpation is frequently required. (See also under 'Mycobacteria' in section on 'Therapy by Pathogen'.)

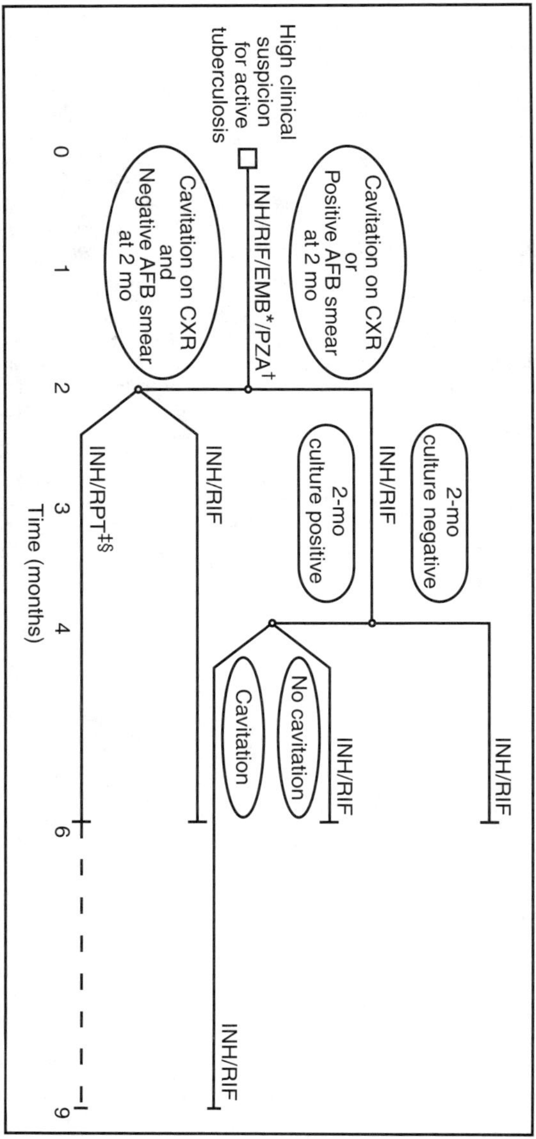

Figure 1: Treatment algorithm for TB in patients with proven or strongly suspected disease. *EMB may be discontinued when results of drug susceptibility testing indicate no drug resistance. †PZA may be discontinued after it has been taken for 2 mo (56 doses). ‡RPT should not be used in HIV-infected patients with TB or in patients with extrapulmonary TB. §Therapy should be extended to 9 mo if 2-mo culture is positive. CXR = chest radiograph; EMB = ethambutol; INH = isoniazid; PZA = pyrazinamide; RIF = rifampin; RPT = rifapentine.

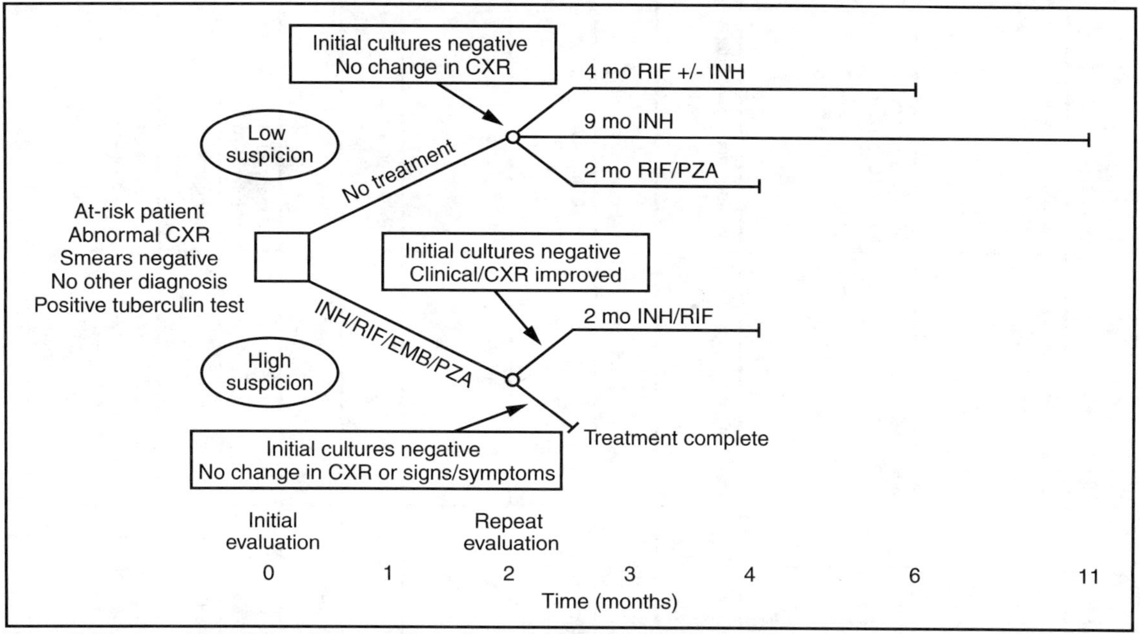

Figure 2: Treatment for active, culture-negative pulmonary TB or inactive TB. *Am J Respir Crit Care Med* 2003;167:602-662.

Tuberculosis *(continued)*

Antituberculosis Therapy

Drug	Usual Adult Dose	Usual Pediatric Dose (after 3 mo of age)
isoniazid (INH)	5 mg/kg/d up to 300 mg in single dose	10-20 mg/kg up to 300 mg/d in single dose
rifampin	600 mg/d, single dose P.O. or IV	10-20 mg/kg/d not to exceed 600 mg/d
ethambutol	15-25 mg/kg/d, single dose	not recommended under age 13
pyrazinamide	P.O. 15-30 mg/kg/d divided into 1-4 doses	15-30 mg/kg/d q 12-24 h* not to exceed 2 g/d
streptomycin	1 g/d IM	20-40 mg/kg/d
p-aminosalicylic acid (PAS)	150 mg/kg/d in 3 doses	150 mg/kg/d in 3 doses
ethionamide	15-20 mg/kg/d	10-20 mg/kg/d in 2-3 doses (see pediatrician)*
cycloserine	0.25-0.5 g q 12 h in 3 doses Do not exceed 1 g/d.	not recommended
kanamycin	1 g/d	15 mg/kg/d not to exceed 1 g
capreomycin	1 g/d	not approved
clofazimine (for *Mycobacterium leprae*)	for dapsone-sensitive and resistant leprosy, 100 mg daily with other anti-leprosy agents for 2-3 yr, followed by monotherapy	safety and efficacy not established

*Not FDA-approved.

Some Common Side Effects/Comments
To be used in conjunction with other agents. Children tolerate INH better. Peripheral neuropathy rare (controlled by pyridoxine 50 mg/d). Central neurologic disorders, rashes, fever. Because fulminant liver failure may occur, all patients should be monitored at least monthly by physicians, and appropriate laboratory tests of liver function should be performed. Black and Hispanic women are at increased risk of toxicity. Monitor alcohol intake.
To be used in conjunction with other agents. Hepatotoxicity; perhaps increased with INH coadministration. Influenzalike syndrome, rash, pruritus, GI, eosinophilia, reversible leukopenia, raised BUN and serum uric acid. Accelerates hepatic inactivation of concurrent medication, eg, methadone, coumarin, estrogens, corticosteroids, theophylline, ketoconazole, and (?) cyclosporine + other cardiovascular agents, digoxin. Serum half-life (h)—normal: 1.5-5.0; oliguria: 3-7.
To be used in conjunction with other agents. Retrobulbar neuritis at higher dosages. Evaluate vision and color perception. Not recommended in children under 13 years of age.
Adverse reactions: GI symptoms, liver toxicity, arthralgia, increases uric acid, rash.
See 'Aminoglycosides.' Must not be sole agent in TB therapy—resistance emerges rapidly. Usually administered with INH for first 3 months in extrapulmonary disease.
To be used in conjunction with other agents. Children tolerate PAS better, GI symptoms frequent in adults—may use resin-coated or purified PAS-C forms. Hypokalemia, leukopenia, hepatitis, fever, goiter, allergic reaction (occasionally severe). Keep PAS in cool, dry place. Rarely used in United States.
Hepatotoxic. GI irritation.
To be used in conjunction with other agents. Neurologic and cerebral side effects, particularly in elderly. Dosage to be monitored by blood levels.
Hypokalemia, hypomagnesemia, ototoxicity, nephrotoxicity
To be used in conjunction with other agents. Electrolyte depletion, raised BUN, urine-albumin, casts, cells. Eighth-nerve damage, fever, eosinophilia, rash.

Antiviral Agents

Burt R. Meyers, MD, FACP

New viruses are constantly being discovered, and old viruses continue to adapt and spread, increasing the chance that they will cause human infection. The development of antiviral agents is ongoing.

West Nile Virus

West Nile virus, a flavivirus, has been reported across the United States. Most infections occur in the summer months. Symptoms include encephalitis and, often, muscle aches and pains; acute flaccid paralysis may occur. Although no therapy has been proven effective, two investigational therapies are available: (1) interferon plus ribavirin, and (2) immunoglobulin. Transfusion-associated West Nile virus has been reported, as well as transmission via solid organs. A vaccine and a monoclonal antibody directed against West Nile virus are being studied.

Avian Influenza Viruses

Avian influenza viruses, mainly H5N1, have been reported, occurring most commonly in Southeast Asia. Ducks and chickens remain the main reservoir. Severe infections have occurred in humans, with an initial death rate of about 70%. Recent serologic analysis of rural populations has reported a low seroprevalence rate, suggesting that subclinical infections may occur. The reported cases have been in rural families who have contact with chickens and ducks. Human-to-human transmission has not been documented but was suggested in one case. The neuraminidase inhibitors oseltamivir and zanamivir are active against avian influenza viruses in vitro. In the autumn of 2004, H7N1 was isolated in a patient in New York State; he recovered and no other cases were reported.

Recently, avian strain H5N1 was isolated in Java, Indonesia.

SARS

Severe acute respiratory syndrome (SARS) associated with a coronavirus (SAR-CoV) that caused infections in Hong Kong and Canada in 2003 seems to have disappeared.

Rabies Virus

The cure of an infected patient who did not receive postexposure prophylaxis has been recently reported. Treatment involved pharmacologic central nervous system depression and use of amantadine and ribavirin. In 2004, rabies transmission from one infected donor led to the death of all solid-organ recipients from that donor.

Antiviral Agents*

Antiviral agents are available in the U.S: three are topical only—trifluridine, idoxuridine, and vidarabine (ara-A); amantadine, valacyclovir, valganciclovir, oseltamivir, zanamivir and famciclovir are oral agents. Acyclovir may be given orally, parenterally, and topically. Ganciclovir is given parenterally and orally and as an eye implant.

Acyclovir (intravenous)

This drug is highly selective because of its affinity for thymidine kinase, found in HSV and varicella zoster virus (VZV). This enzyme converts acyclovir to acyclovir monophosphate and further converts it into a triphosphate. Acyclovir triphosphate stops viral replication of herpesvirus DNA, including inactivation of viral DNA polymerase. Acyclovir is more active against HSV than against VZV because of more efficient phosphorylation by thymidine kinase.

Pharmacokinetics: The $T½$ is 2.5-3.3 h. Oral bioavailability is 10% to 20%; no effect of food. Plasma protein binding is 9%-33%. C_{max} at 200 mg = 0.83 µg/mL; at 400 mg = 1.2 µg/mL; and at 800 mg = 1.61 µg/mL.

Indications and Dosage:

- **HSV-1 and HSV-2 mucosal and cutaneous infection in immunocompromised patients:** adults and children aged 12 years and older, 5 mg/kg (given over 1 h) q 8 h x 7 days; pediatric dose (younger than 12 years), 10 mg/kg (given over 1 h) q 8 h x 7 days.
- **Severe initial herpes genitalis in adults and children aged 12 years and older:** 5 mg/kg (given over 1 h) q 8 h x 5 days. For herpes simplex encephalitis: adults and children aged 12 years and older, 10 mg/kg (infused over 1 h) q 8 h x 10 days; pediatric dose (younger than 12 years), 20 mg/kg (infused slowly over 1 h) q 8 h x 10 days.
- **Varicella zoster in immunocompromised patients:** adults and children aged 12 years and older, 10 mg/kg (infused over 1 h) q 8 h x 7 days; pediatric dose (younger than 12 years), 20 mg/kg (infused over 1 h) q 8 h x 7 days. For patients with impaired renal function, see Table 4, Section 17.

Side Effects: Phlebitis, transient elevations of serum creatinine, rash; rarely, diaphoresis, hematuria, hypotension, headache, nausea, and CNS toxicity. Avoid rapid or bolus injection.

Acyclovir (oral)

Dosage: 200 mg q 4 h (5 doses per day for herpes simplex infection) for 10 days for total of 50 capsules. Dosage for varicella zoster is 800 mg given 5 times per day for 7 to 10 days.

- **Chronic suppressive therapy:** Acyclovir 400 mg b.i.d. x 12 months has been given to prevent recurrences of herpes simplex infections.

Other suppressive regimens are 200 mg either 3 or 5 times daily.

- **Intermittent therapy:** 200 mg q 4 h 5 times daily for 5 days initiated at earliest symptoms (prodrome) of recurrence.

For treatment of chickenpox at age 2 years and older: 20 mg/kg/dose 4 times daily (80 mg/kg/day). Children >40 kg get an adult dose. The adult dose is 800 mg 4 times daily for 5 days. For acute and chronic renal impairment: see Table 5, Section 17. For hemodialysis: Administer an additional dose after each dialysis. No supplemental dosing for peritoneal dialysis.

Side Effects: Nausea and/or vomiting; diarrhea; malaise. CNS changes more commonly seen with IV formulation, but may be marked, especially in older patients with renal impairment.

Safety and Efficacy: Safety and efficacy of orally administered acyclovir as treatment for the suppression of recurrent episodes of genital herpes have been established only for up to 12 months, although some patients have taken the drug for up to 10 years (not FDA approved for this length of therapy).

*Not including antivirals active against HIV.

Acyclovir Ointment 5%

Topical preparation indicated for the management of initial herpes genitalis in immunocompetent patients, and for the treatment of limited mucocutaneous herpes simplex virus infections in immunocompromised patients.

Route: Topical application; use of a finger cot or rubber glove is recommended to prevent autoinoculation of other body sites and transmission of infection to other persons.

Dosage and Duration: The ointment should be applied 6 times a day for 7 days. Therapy should be initiated as early as possible after onset of signs and symptoms.

Side Effects: Patients may experience mild burning when ointment is applied. In all studies, there was no significant difference between the drug and placebo group in the rate or type of reported adverse reactions.

Valacyclovir

A more bioavailable form of acyclovir, indicated for the treatment of herpes zoster and the treatment of suppression of genital herpes. The drug relieves acute signs, symptoms, and duration of postherpetic neuralgia. Indicated for initial and recurrent genital herpes.

Route: Oral.

Dosage: For herpes zoster: 1 g given t.i.d. for 7 days; for initial genital herpes: 1 g b.i.d. for 10 days; for recurrent genital herpes: 500 mg b.i.d. x 5 days. For suppression of genital herpes: 500 mg once daily for up to 8 months. For cold sores: 2 g x 2 doses 12 h apart (1-day treatment). Drug should be initiated within 72 hours of rash onset. Reduction adjustment in renal failure and in geriatric patients with reduced renal function (see Tables 13 and 14, Section 17).

Drug/Drug Interactions: Cimetidine and probenecid increase drug levels of acyclovir.

Side Effects: Nausea, headache, vomiting.

Note: Thrombotic thrombocytopenic purpura/hemolytic uremic syndrome (TTP/HUS), in some cases resulting in death, has occurred in patients with advanced HIV disease and also in allogeneic bone marrow transplant and renal transplant recipients in clinical trials of valacyclovir at doses of 8 g/d. This was not observed in clinical trials in immunocompetent patients.

Ganciclovir

A synthetic guanine derivative active against CMV and HSV. To be active, ganciclovir is phosphorylated to a monophosphate form by a CMV encoded gene (VL97) protein kinase analogue, then to diphosphate and triphosphate forms by cellular kinases. The triphosphate form has 100 times greater concentration in cells infected with CMV and inhibits viral DNA synthesis by competitive inhibition of viral DNA polymerase and by terminating viral DNA prolongation.

Route: P.O., IV.

Pharmacology: Poorly bioavailable, 5% to 9% (with food), with 86% recovered in feces. Ganciclovir achieves cerebrospinal fluid (CSF) concentrations of 0.31 to 0.68 μg/mL. Plasma protein binding is 1%-2%. Following IV administration, 91% is recovered in urine. The $T\frac{1}{2}$ is 3.5 h following IV administration and 4.8 h following oral administration.

Indications: IV ganciclovir is indicated for CMV retinitis and prophylaxis of CMV in transplant patients. Oral ganciclovir is indicated for prevention of CMV in transplant and HIV-infected patients and for maintenance therapy of CMV retinitis after IV therapy.

Dosage/Treatment: The following doses are for patients with normal renal function.

- **Induction therapy of CMV retinitis:** 5 mg/kg (IV) for 1 h q 12 h x 14-21 days.
- **Maintenance therapy:** 1,000 mg t.i.d. orally with food.

• **Prevention of CMV retinitis in HIV-infected patients:** 1,000 mg t.i.d. with food.

• **Prevention of CMV disease in transplant patients:** 5 mg/kg q 12 h for 7-14 days followed by 5 mg/kg q 24 h daily *or* 6 mg/kg q 24 h x 5 days per week.

• **Oral ganciclovir for prevention of CMV:** 1,000 mg/kg t.i.d. with food.

Length of treatment is based on clinical status. In some bone marrow transplant trials, ganciclovir was given for 100-120 days post-transplantation. For renal insufficiency, see Table 6 in Section 17.

Adverse Events: Granulocytopenia, anemia, and thrombocytopenia. Drug is contraindicated if neutrophil count is <500 cells/μL or platelet count is <25,000 cells/μL. Affects spermatogenesis; drug is embryotoxic in rabbits and carcinogenic in a mouse model. Not known whether drug is excreted in breast milk, so should not be used by nursing mothers. Safety and efficacy not known in pediatric patients. Use only with extreme caution because there is a probability of long-term carcinogenesis and reproductive toxicity.

Valganciclovir

An L-valyl-ester (prodrug) of ganciclovir. The bioavailability is 60% with food. When taken orally, the drug is rapidly metabolized to ganciclovir, and the pharmacokinetics are similar to those described above. The $T\frac{1}{2}$ is 4-6.8 h. Toxicity is similar to that of ganciclovir.

Indications: Valganciclovir is indicated for prevention of CMV disease in kidney, kidney/pancreas, and heart transplant patients at high risk (D+ R-) and for treatment of CMV retinitis in HIV patients. Not indicated for prophylaxis in liver transplants.

Route: P.O.

Dosage:

• **Transplant patients with normal renal function:** 900 mg b.i.d. starting 10 days before transplantation and continuing 100 days post-transplant.

• **Induction therapy of CMV retinitis:** 900 mg b.i.d. with food for 21 days, then 900 mg q.d. with food.

For patients with renal insufficiency, see Table 7 in Section 17.

Foscarnet

An antiviral agent that inhibits replication of herpes virus in vitro, including cytomegalovirus (CMV) and herpes simplex virus types 1 and 2 (HSV-1, HSV-2). The mode of action is on virus-specific DNA polymerases at concentrations that do not affect cellular DNA polymerases. Foscarnet does not require phosphorylation by thymidine kinase or other kinases and therefore is active in vitro against HSV TK-deficient mutants and CMV VL97 mutants.

Foscarnet is active against most CMV strains resistant to ganciclovir and acyclovir. However, if acyclovir or ganciclovir resistance is due to alterations in viral DNA polymerase, foscarnet will not be active. Combination of foscarnet and ganciclovir has enhanced activity in vitro.

Route: IV.

Pharmacokinetics: After IV administration: $T\frac{1}{2}$ is 4 hours in plasma; 14% to 17% is protein bound. The drug is renally cleared but accumulates in bone. In patients with decreased renal function, the $T\frac{1}{2}$ may be 25 h.

Indications: Foscarnet is indicated for treatment only in immunocompromised patients with CMV retinitis and mucocutaneous, acyclovir-resistant HSV infections.

Dosage and Administration: All patients' renal function must be monitored. Patients should be hydrated, which may reduce risk of toxicity. Administering 750-1,000 mL of normal saline is recommended before first dose. (Follow-up hydration depends on dosage selected.) **Caution:** IV drugs **must not** be given by rapid bolus injection.

• **Normal renal function—induction:** For patients with CMV retinitis, either 90 mg/kg ($1\frac{1}{2}$ to 2 h infusion) q 12 h or 60 mg/kg (1 h infusion) q 8 h over 2-3 weeks, depending on response. For acyclovir-resistant HSV, 40 mg/kg (1 h infusion) q 8-12 h for 2-3 weeks or until lesion heals.

• **Normal renal function—maintenance:** For CMV retinitis, 90-120 mg/kg/day (adjusted for renal function) over 2 h. Infusion pump is required to control rate of infusion, hydration is recommended. Patients with progression of retinitis may receive combination of foscarnet and ganciclovir (**not** in same IV mixture).

• **Abnormal renal function:** Foscarnet should be used with caution in patients with abnormal renal function. Serum levels will be increased, and foscarnet can further impair renal function. For dosage, see Table 15, Section 17. If creatine clearance falls below 0.4 mL/min/kg, drug should be discontinued and patients carefully hydrated and monitored.

Adverse Reactions/Toxicity: Renal impairment is main toxicity; seizures related to plasma mineral and electrolyte concentrations, impaired renal function, and underlying CNS abnormalities. This is probably secondary to chelation of divalent cations (eg, calcium). Perioral tingling, numbness, and paresthesia may occur. Careful management of electrolyte levels is necessary. Anemia and granulocytopenia have been reported. No data exist on use in pregnancy, and it is not known whether drug is found in human milk. Safety and efficacy in children have not been established. Deposition in bone occurs and may be greater in developing bone in children.

Drug Interactions: Foscarnet and pentamidine may have caused hypocalcemia. Foscarnet should be avoided in combination with other nephrotoxic drugs (eg, aminoglycosides, amphotericin B) and pentamidine unless potential benefits outweigh risks.

Famciclovir

A new antiviral agent and prodrug analogue of penciclovir. Indicated for the management of acute herpes zoster. The drug relieves acute signs, symptoms, and duration of postherpetic neuralgia. Indicated for treatment of recurrent genital herpes, when administered within 6 hours of onset. Because 94% of the drug is excreted in the urine, dosage adjustments are necessary in patients with renal dysfunction. The compound does not affect the P-450 enzyme system.

Achieves higher intracellular levels than acyclovir and has a longer intracellular half-life, but the clinical significance of this is unknown.

Route: Oral.

Dosage and Duration: For genital herpes: 125 mg every 12 h x 5 days. For herpes zoster: 500 mg q 8 h x 7 days. Drug should be initiated within 72 hours of rash onset.

Pharmacology: May be taken with meals. Theophylline and digoxin levels increased when coadministered. Increased famciclovir drug levels when given with cimetidine.

Side Effects: Headache, nausea, fatigue.

Dosage Adjustment: Necessary with renal insufficiency (see Table 12, Section 17).

Amantadine

Prophylactic and early therapeutic oral agent against infection with influenza virus (A strains). Must be taken orally, b.i.d., for entire period of possible exposure to influenza virus. Causes transient CNS side effects. Use for hospitalized patients during an epidemic, or as an alternative or supplement to vaccine for high-risk persons during a community epidemic. Contraindicated in pregnant women and nursing mothers. Organisms inhibited: Influenza A, all strains. **Note: Amantadine is not active against avian influenza strains (eg, H5N1, H7N7).**

Route: P.O.

Dose: 100 mg, b.i.d. (adult dosage).

Duration: Entire period during exposure.

Side Effects: Dizziness, drowsiness, convulsions, hallucinations, psychosis; more prominent in middle-aged and elderly individuals.

Rimantadine

An antiviral agent that is believed to inhibit early viral replication, possibly inhibiting uncoating of the virus. The drug is active against influenza A strains, including H1N1, H2N2, and H3N2. It is available orally and is extensively metabolized by the liver, with 25% of drug excreted unchanged in urine. It is not recommended in pregnancy and is contraindicated for nursing mothers. Pharmacokinetics parameters following a 100-mg dose revealed a C_{max} of 74 ng/mL and a $T\frac{1}{2}$ of 25.4 h (32 h in healthy elderly subjects aged 71-79 years). **Note: Rimantadine is not active against avian influenza strains (eg, H5N1, H7N7).**

Route: P.O.

Dosage:

- **For prophylaxis:** 100 mg b.i.d. (elderly, 100 mg q.d.); in children younger than 10 years, 5 mg/kg/day (not to exceed 150 mg).
- **Therapy in adults:** Continue 7 days from initial onset of symptoms with dose of 100 mg b.i.d.; in elderly nursing home residents, 100 mg q.d. Use with caution in patients with reduced renal clearance and hepatic insufficiency.

Side Effects: Dizziness, insomnia, GI symptoms (less severe than with amantadine).

Drug/Drug Interactions: Aspirin and acetaminophen reduce peak plasma level of rimantadine by ~10%. Cimetidine reduced clearance of rimantadine by 18%.

Oseltamivir

An antiviral agent that inhibits influenza virus neuraminidase, oseltamivir is an ester requiring hydrolysis for conversion to the active form, oseltamivir carboxylate. The drug is given orally, with 75% reaching the bloodstream in the active state; food does not affect absorption; and 99% of the active drug is renally excreted. The $T\frac{1}{2}$ is 1-3 h. Protein binding of active compound is low (3%). Drug is neither substrate nor inhibitor of cytochrome P450 isoforms. Peak concentrations are 441-457 ng/mL. No dosage adjustments for elderly patients for either prophylaxis or treatment.

Route: P.O.

Indications: Prophylaxis and treatment of influenza.

Dosage:

- **Treatment of adults:** 75 mg b.i.d. x 5 days, begun within 2 days of onset of symptoms.
- **Pediatric patients older than 1 year:** Varies by weight.

<15 kg = 30 mg b.i.d.
>15-23 kg = 45 mg b.i.d.
23-40 kg = 60 mg b.i.d.
>40 kg = 75 kg b.i.d.

Dosage adjustment for creatine clearance 10-30 mL/min: To 75 mg q.d.

- **Prophylaxis in adults and children older than 13 years who had contact with infected individuals:** 75 mg q.d. x 7 days. Therapy should begin within 2 days of exposure. In a community outbreak, the dose is 75 mg q.d. Protection lasts as long as the drug is taken. Dosage adjustment for creatine clearance 10-30 mL/mg: To 75 mg q.o.d. *or* 30 mg oral suspension q.d.

Pregnancy: In pregnancy and lactation, the recommendation is for use only if potential benefits justify the risk to fetus or nursing infant.

Side Effects: Nausea, vomiting, and diarrhea are most common and usually occur during the first 2 days.

Drug/Drug Interactions: Insignificant.

Note: In vitro oseltamivir is active against avian influenza strains (eg, H5N1, H7N7).

Zanamivir

Antiviral agent that inhibits influenza virus neuraminidase. After inhalation, 4% to 17% of inhaled dose is absorbed systemically. Peak serum concentrations are 17-142 ng/mL within 1-2 hours following 10 mg dose. Plasma protein binding is less than 10%. The drug is renally excreted, with no metabolites detected in humans. The T½ is 2.5-5.1 h. Drug interactions are not significant. **In vitro drug is active against avian influenza strains, including H5N1 and H7N7.**

Route: Inhalation.

Indications: Treatment of uncomplicated acute influenza caused by influenza A or B in adults and children aged 7 years and older who have had symptoms for no more than 2 days. Not recommended for patients with asthma or chronic obstructive pulmonary disease.

Dosage: Two inhalations (one 5 mg blister per inhalation for a total of 10 mg) b.i.d. If using a bronchodilator, administer before taking zanamivir. **Note:** Patients need to be instructed on use of the delivery system.

Side Effects: Bronchospasm and decrease in lung function. Zanamivir is not recommended in patients with underlying airway disease.

Studies: The drug has not been studied in patients with impaired hepatic function, patients older than 65 years, or patients with severe renal insufficiency.

Pregnancy: Recommendation is that zanamivir only be used when potential benefit justifies potential risk to the fetus. It is not known whether zanamivir is present in human milk, so caution is necessary if administered to nursing mothers.

Note: In vitro drug is active against avian influenza strains, including H5N1 and H7N1.

Trifluridine Solution

Indicated for treatment of primary keratoconjunctivitis and recurrent epithelial keratitis due to herpes simplex virus, types 1 and 2. Trifluridine was found to be effective in 138 of 150 patients unresponsive or intolerant to idoxuridine or vidarabine. Available in solution form, trifluridine requires fewer applications, with no nighttime dosage and none of the blurring and inconveniences of ointments.

Dosage: One drop every 2 h while awake until lesion has completely re-epithelialized, then one drop every 4 h for 7 days thereafter.

Adverse Reactions: Burning or stinging upon instillation (less than 5%) and palpebral edema (less than 3%) were noted in controlled clinical trials.

Idoxuridine (IDU)

Indicated for herpes simplex keratitis (acute and superficial disease). Not for stromal involvement. Does not prevent recurrence.

The Antifungals

Jack D. Sobel, MD

Despite the increased availability of a wider selection of antifungal agents, invasive fungal disease continues to represent a major health threat, particularly in immunocompromised patients. Significant changes have occurred in overall epidemiology. For the first time in many decades, the number of candidemia episodes in the United States has declined. Moreover, the prevalence of most cases has shifted from units catering to patients with hematologic malignancies and neutropenia to medical and surgical intensive care units. In addition, the mortality of candidemia cases has declined, primarily because of the increased awareness and willingness of practitioners to treat *all* cases of candidemia. There had been a trend to only observe patients with transient candidemia. Now all patients with invasive candidiasis, including candidemia, should be treated.

The episodes of candidemia have also decreased among oncology patients, a consequence of the widespread use of fluconazole prophylaxis. Accordingly, the epicenter of invasive *Candida* disease is now reflected in critically ill medical and surgical patients, including neonates, and is primarily a result of intravascular cather-related infections. At the same time, mold infections have increased in immunocompromised cancer patients, and more unusual molds are occurring, as well as aspergillosis. The increased occurrence of *Zygomyces* is a concern.

Since the last edition of this book, there have been several changes in the availability and use of antifungal agents. A national trend has emerged to use less amphotericin B deoxycholate. Accordingly, conventional amphotericin B is used far less frequently because of its predictable, inevitable, and virtually unavoidable toxicity and side effects. In part, the slack has been picked up by the use of the lipid formulations of amphotericin B. Newer azoles and echinocandins have become available. Fluconazole, which was the workhorse of yeast infections, has become generic. Accordingly, both oral and parenteral fluconazole are available at significant cost savings, so this drug remains the cornerstone of the management and prevention of fungal infections.

In the last 2 years, voriconazole, a new-generation triazole, has emerged as the drug of first choice for the treatment of invasive aspergillosis. It has also has proved very useful in the treatment of previously resistant mold infections, including *Fusarium* and *Scedosporium* infections. Although also approved for the treatment of esophageal candidiasis, as well as candidemia and invasive candidiasis, there is little evidence that voriconazole offers a major advantage for these yeast infections unless resistant species are involved, such as *Candida krusei* and the rarely resistant *Candida albicans*. Accordingly, voriconazole has proven particularly useful in the management of mold infections. In clinical practice, it is now common to use voriconazole in combination with an echinocandin, particularly for severe forms of aspergillosis. Because little scientific data exist to support combination antifungal use for this indication, there is a critical need for prospective studies evaluating combination antifungal therapy.

A trend that has prompted concern with voriconazole is its frequent, unapproved use as long-term prophylaxis in bone marrow transplant recipients. In these patients, mold infections such as *Zygomyces* as well as breakthrough *Candida glabrata* infections have emerged.

The single biggest change in antifungals in the last few years has been the availability of the echinocandins. Caspofungin, the first approved echinocandin, has enjoyed major success as first-line therapy for the treatment of invasive candidiasis. The advantages of caspofungin include its broad spectrum, its relatively few drug interactions, and its tolerance in patients with renal failure. Caspofungin has been approved as a secondary drug for refractory aspergillosis, although clinical practice indicates that it is used commonly in combination with voriconazole. More recently, micafungin has been approved for the treatment of esophageal candidiasis and as prophylaxis of *Candida* infections in neutropenic patients. Yet another echinocandin, anidulafungin, is expected to be approved in 2005 for invasive candidiasis. The echinocandins are likely to dominate the treatment of *Candida* infections, and their role in combination therapy should be determined by prospective studies. Posaconazole, an experimental triazole, has proved useful in case series for the treatment of life-threatening *Zygomyces* infections.

The Antifungals *(continued)*

Amphotericin B: Polyene antibiotic inhibits cryptococci, *Candida, Sporotrichum, Blastomyces, Paracoccidioides, Histoplasma, Coccidioides, Aspergillus, Naegleria*. Acts synergistically with 5-fluorocytosine. Not absorbed orally, must be given by IV route, stable to light for 8 h. Renal-toxic, arrhythmias if given rapidly, allergic reactions, fever, hypotension, liver function test abnormalities, hypokalemia.

Amphotericin B Lipid Complex: New formulation that allows higher dosing of amphotericin, ie, 5 mg/kg; it appears to be less nephrotoxic. Indicated for treatment of invasive fungal infections in patients refractory to or intolerant of conventional amphotericin B therapy.

Amphotericin B Liposome: Another agent released for the treatment of refractory fungal infections and visceral leishmaniasis.

5-Flucytosine (5-fluorocytosine): Inhibits cryptococci and some yeast *Candida* species, including *C glabrata*. Resistance of yeast develops rapidly. Should usually be used with amphotericin B. Absorbed orally, renally excreted, accumulates in renal failure. Causes nausea, diarrhea, converted in gut to 5-fluorouracil, causes hepatotoxicity and bone marrow depression.

Clotrimazole: Imidazole inhibits dermatophytes, molds such as *Aspergillus, Penicillium*, cryptococci, *Candida*, and dimorphic fungi such as *Sporotrichum* and *Coccidioides*. Only topically.

Drug	Organisms Inhibited	Route	Dose
amphotericin B	*Aspergillus, Candida, Blastomyces, Coccidioides*, cryptococci, *Histoplasma Phycomycetes, Paracoccidioides, Sporotrichum, Leishmania*	IV irrigation	0.6-1.0 mg/kg/d 5 mg, variable
nystatin	as above	P.O. vaginal inserts	10^4 u-10^6 u q 6 h apply q.d.
pimaricin	as above	eye solution	every 2-4 h x 3-4 d then q 3-4 h for a total of 14-21 d
5-flucytosine	cryptococci, *Candida*, including *C glabrata, Chromoblastomyces*	P.O.	150 mg/kg/d in 3-4 doses
clotrimazole	dermatophytes, molds, cryptococci, *Candida*	topical vaginal	b.i.d. qhs

Fluconazole: Triazole with activity against cryptococci, *Candida* species, *Blastomyces*, and *Histoplasma*. T½ of 30 hours allows once-daily dosing. Effective in treating oral and esophageal candidiasis, *Candida* urinary tract infections, peritonitis, and systemic *Candida* infections, including candidemia, disseminated candidiasis, and vaginal candidiasis. Useful for prophylaxis in patients undergoing bone marrow transplantation receiving chemotherapy and/or radiation therapy. Available in oral suspension, IV, and tablets.

Miconazole: Imidazole inhibits cryptococci, *Candida*, *Coccidioides*, and *Pseudallescheria boydii* (resistant to amphotericin B). For topical or intravenous use in superficial infections. No longer used or available for parenteral use.

Ketoconazole: Synthetic antifungal agent with broad spectrum. Active in vitro against dermatophytes, *Candida*, *Histoplasma*, *Blastomyces*, *Coccidioides immitis*, and cryptococci. Long half-life; 99% protein binding. Drug impairs fungal cell membrane synthesis. Has been used successfully in some systemic fungal infections, ie, candidiasis, candiduria, histoplasmosis, paracoccidioidomycosis. Penetrates poorly into CSF and should not be used for meningitis. May decrease cortisol and other androgenic hormones. Severe hepatotoxicity may occur, including fatalities. There is a risk of developing life-threatening arrhythmias if used with terfenadine, so these drugs should not be given together. Astemizole is

Serum T½			
Normal	**Oliguria**	**Duration**	**Common Side Effects/Comments**
24 h	24 h	unknown 1-2 g empiric	Minor renal excretion. Rapid infusion produces hypotension. Fever, arrhythmias, hypokalemia, increased SGOT, anemia, azotemia common. Reversible blood dyscrasias. Soluble only in water—comes out of solution in saline. Avoid reactions by pretreating with either salicylates, antihistamines, or hydrocortisone. Daily dose depends on indication; 0.4-1.0 mg/kg/d.
–	–	while on antibiotics 7-10 d	Use in immunosuppressed patients and in patients on long-term broad-spectrum antibiotics. Rarely used today.
–	–	while infection persists	Effective in superficial fungal keratoses and postoperative fungal eye infections.
5 h	60 h	unknown	Coadminister with amphotericin B to obtain synergy. Leukopenia, diarrhea. Adjust dose in renal failure. Useful for candiduria, especially in presence of non-albicans *Candida*.
–	–	7-10 d	Very effective in mixed *Candida*-dermatophyte infections.

continued on next page

The Antifungals *(continued)*

also contraindicated. Because of possible multiple drug interactions, see package insert before prescribing. Not available parenterally, only orally. Given its toxicity, ketoconazole is rarely used today.

Itraconazole: Synthetic triazole antifungal agent available in oral and IV forms with broad antifungal activity, including *Candida* sp, *Aspergillus* sp, cryptococci, *Histoplasma* sp, etc. Released for the treatment of pulmonary and extrapulmonary blastomycosis and histoplasmosis, chronic, cavitary and disseminated (not for meningeal).

Drug	Organisms Inhibited	Route	Dose
ketoconazole	dermatophytes, *Candida, Histoplasma, Blastomyces, Coccidioides immitis,* cryptococci	P.O.	200 mg/d; serious infections 400 mg/d
miconazole	dermatophytes, cryptococci, *Candida, Coccidioides, Pseudallescheria boydii*	topical 2%	apply topically PRN
griseofulvin	dermatophytes	P.O.	Adults: 0.5-1.0 g/d
terconazole	vulvovaginal candidiasis	vaginal suppository	once daily HS x 3 d
fluconazole	*Candida* sp cryptococci	P.O. IV oral suspension	Adults: candidal UTI: 50-200 mg/d (see package insert for pediatric equivalents) systemic infection: up to 400 mg/d
	Candida sp	P.O.	Esophageal and/or oropharyngal candidiasis: suspension 200 mg day 1, then 100 mg/d Vaginal candidiasis: 150 mg single oral dose tablet

Voriconazole: A triazole agent available both P.O. and IV, with excellent activity against *Aspergillus* species and other fungi such as *Scedosporium* and *Fusarium* in patients intolerant to other antifungals. Also has in vitro activity against *Candida* species. Has numerous drug interactions and is contraindicated in the presence of rifampin.

Caspofungin acetate: A new class of antifungal drugs (echinocandins) that inhibits glucan synthesis, a part of the fungal cell wall, and is active against *Aspergillus* and *Candida* species. Caspofungin is indicated for the treatment of invasive aspergillosis in patients who are refractory or intolerant to other therapies, such as amphoteri-

Serum T½			
Normal	**Oliguria**	**Duration**	**Common Side Effects/Comments**
Biphasic: 2 for 1st 10 h, then 8	27 h	variable	Hepatotoxicity may be fatal; must monitor hepatic function. Poor diffusion into CSF. (For disease indications, see package insert.) May affect cortisol secretion. Terfenadine, astemizole, and cisapride are contraindicated. Triazolam levels may be increased.
—	—	while infection persists 7-10 d	Liver, lipoprotein, CNS effects. Failures of cryptococcosis and coccidioidomycosis. Cisapride is contraindicated. Not recommended as IV because of arrhythmias.
12 h	12 h	variable, 2-8 wk	Follow liver enzymes; alters anticoagulation, rashes.
			Cisapride is contraindicated. Influenza-like syndrome is reported.
30 h	increased	14-28 d 10-12 wk for cryptococcal meningitis	Drug/drug interactions: Fluconazole levels cause enhanced activity of anticoagulant and hypoglycemic agents, and increased levels of cyclosporine and phenytoin. Rifampin may decrease levels of fluconazole. Cisapride and terfenadine are contraindicated. Maintenance Rx given for cryptococcal meningitis. Triazolam levels may be increased.

continued on next page

The Antifungals *(continued)*

cin B and/or lipid formulations, and itraconazole. Its main use is as first-line therapy for candidemia and invasive candidiasis. Its use is not recommended with cyclosporine. Caspofungin does not induce the P-450 cytochrome system. However, coadministration with inducer/inhibitor drugs (such as some AIDS drugs), rifampin, phenytoin, and dexamethasone may require an increase in the daily dose. While no dose adjustment is necessary for renal insufficiency, the dose should be lowered for those with moderate hepatic insufficiency. Side effects include possible histamine-mediated symptoms, including facial swelling and pruritus.

Drug	Organisms Inhibited	Route	Dose
itraconazole	*Histoplasma** *Blastomyces** *Aspergillus***	P.O. or IV	200-400 mg q.d. x 3 mo 200 mg q.d. x 3 mo 200-400 mg q.d. x 3 mo
	candidiasis	IV or P.O. Solution (not recommended as initial therapy)	Esophageal: 100 mg swished in mouth q.d. x 3 wk Oropharyngeal: 200 mg swished in mouth q.d. x 1-2 wk
		P.O.	Vaginal: 200 mg x 3 d
	sporotrichosis	P.O.	200-400 mg q.d.
	pityriasis versicolor	P.O.	400 mg x 1 dose, or up to 200 mg q.d. x 5-7 d
	onychomycosis	P.O.	
	–fingernail		200 mg b.i.d. x 1 wk, then wait 3 wk and repeat therapy
	–toenail		400 mg q.d. x 1 wk, wait 3 wk and repeat therapy, then wait 3 more wk and repeat therapy again, or 200 mg q.d. x 3 mo
	Capsules should not be administered for treatment of onychomycosis in patients with ventricular dysfunction, such as congestive heart failure (CHF) or a history of CHF.		

* FDA indications

** Pulmonary and extrapulmonary aspergillosis in patients who are intolerant of or refractory to amphotericin B therapy.

Griseofulvin: For oral use, interferes with DNA metabolism, inhibits *Microsporum, Epidermophyton, Trichophyton.* No effect on other fungi. Side effects: nausea, diarrhea, rash, headaches. Interferes with porphyrin metabolism, reduces anticoagulant effect.
Nystatin: For topical use. Inhibits yeasts and molds. Resistance can develop. Side effects are rare.

Tolnaftate: For topical use. Effective against dermatophytes, *Trichophyton, Microsporum, Epidermophyton.* No effect on *Candida.* Most useful in skin infections, less so in hair and nail infections.
Haloprogin: Phenolic ether for topic use. Effective against *Epidermophyton, Microsporum, Trichophyton,* and *Candida.* Inhibits O_2 uptake in fungi. Resistance develops. Side effect: occasional rash.

Serum T½ Normal	Serum T½ Oliguria	Duration	Common Side Effects/Comments
21-64 h	–	3 mo	Drug/drug interactions* may occur: Levels of digoxin and cyclosporine increase, as does anticoagulant activity; itraconazole levels decrease with INH, phenytoin, rifampin, H_2-agonists. Oral hyperglycemic activity increases.
35.4 h	–	3 mo	Clarithromycin, indinavir, and ritonavir increase itraconazole levels.
		3 mo	Potent inhibitor of P-450 3A4 enzyme system. Monitor liver function tests in patients with hepatic impairment. Use caution with erythromycin, which may increase levels of itraconazole. **Negative inotropic effects seen in healthy volunteers when given IV dosing. If congestive heart failure occurs, reassess use of itraconazole.**

* See package insert for further drug/drug interactions.

continued on next page

The Antifungals *(continued)*

Drug	Organisms Inhibited	Route	Dose
itraconazole *(continued)*	aspergillosis	IV	200 mg b.i.d. x 4 d, then 200 mg q.d. up to 3 mo
	blastomycosis	IV	200 mg b.i.d. x 4 d, then 200 mg q.d. up to 3 mo
	histoplasmosis	IV	200 mg b.i.d. x 4 d, then 200 mg q.d. up to 3 mo
	Empiric therapy of febrile neutropenic patients with suspected fungal infections	IV	200 mg b.i.d. x 4 d then 200 mg q.d. up to 3 mo

Serum $T^{1}/_{2}$ Normal	Oliguria	Duration	Common Side Effects/Comments
			Ergot alkaloids are contraindicated. **Contraindicated with:** astemizole, dofetilide, terfenadine, cisapride, midazolam, pimozide, quinidine, levacetylmethadol (levomethadyl), or triazolam. **Serious cardiac events, including sudden death, have occurred in patients using many of these drugs with itraconazole. See package insert for full explanation of contraindications.**

continued on next page

The Antifungals *(continued)*

Drug	Organisms Inhibited	Route	Dose
voriconazole	*A fumigatus*, other *Aspergillus* sp, *Scedosporium* sp, *Fusarium*	IV or P.O.	IV: 6 mg/kg q 12 h x 2 doses followed by 4 mg/kg q 12 h then:
	Candida sp	IV or P.O.	P.O.: 200 mg q 12 h if weight >40 kg; if weight is <40 kg, then 100 mg q 12 h

Serum $T^{1/2}$ Normal	Oliguria	Duration	Common Side Effects/Comments
dose dependent	no change	empiric, based on clinical response/ immune restoration, other factors	Oral bioavailability 96%. Hepatic toxicity noted. Visual disturbances, including blurring and photophobia. Monitor hepatic function. Metabolized by P-450 enzymes. Dose adjustments in renal insufficiency may be necessary because of accumulation of vehicle used in IV preparation. No dose change for P.O. in renal insufficiency. Dose adjustments necessary in patients with hepatic insufficiency. Contraindicated with: rifampin, rifabutin, long-acting barbiturates, carbamazepine, cimetidine, sirolimus, ergot alkaloids, terfenadine, astemizole, cisapride, pimozide, quinidine. Will need to reduce dose of tacrolimus to one third and cyclosporine to one half. Adjust dose downward with: warfarin, oral coumarin, statins, calcium channel blockers, benzodiazepines, sulfonylureas, omeprazole. Increase dose of voriconazole to 5 mg/kg q 12 h if patient is receiving phenytoin. Other drugs have mixed effects: see full package insert.

continued on next page

The Antifungals *(continued)*

Drug	Organisms Inhibited	Route	Dose
caspofungin	*Candida* species, *Aspergillus* species* including triazole-resistant strains	IV	70 mg q.d. x 1, then 50 mg q.d.

* Indicated for the treatment of invasive aspergillosis in patients who are refractory to or intolerant of other therapies, ie, amphotericin B, lipid formulations of amphotericin B, and itraconazole. Also indicated for candidemia and invasive candidiasis and as empiric therapy for febrile neutropenic subjects.

Serum $T_{1/2}$ Normal	Serum $T_{1/2}$ Oliguria	Duration	Common Side Effects/Comments
9-11 h	9-11 h	until clinical response	Not active against cryptococci. Adverse reactions include possible histamine-mediated rash, facial swelling, pruritus. No dose adjustment for renal failure; drug is not dialyzable, so no supplementary dosing required after dialysis. Does not inhibit the P-450 cytochrome system, but may decrease tacrolimus levels; increases in ALT/AST noted with cyclosporine, so not recommended. When using efavirenz, nelfinavir, nevirapine, phenytoin, rifampin, dexamethasone, or carbamazepine, may need to increase dose of caspofungin to 70 mg/d. Reduce dose in patients with moderate hepatic insufficiency (Child-Pugh score 7-9) to 35 mg/d after initial dose.

Common Parasitic Infections and Treatment*

Parasite	Drug	Dose (Adult)
Amoeba (intestinal and/or liver abscess)	metronidazole	adult 750 mg P.O. t.i.d. x 10 d treatment should be followed by iodoquinol 650 mg t.i.d. P.O. x 20 d or paromomycin 25-30 mg/kg/q.d. in t.i.d. dosing x 7 d
Ascaris and hookworm (*Ancyclostoma duodenale*/ Necator *americanus*)	mebendazole or albendazole pyrantel pamoate	100 mg b.i.d. P.O. x 3 d or 500 mg P.O. x 1 dose 400 mg P.O. x 1 dose 11 mg/kg x 1 dose
Babesia microti	clindamycin plus quinine**	1.2 g b.i.d. IV or 600 mg t.i.d. P.O. x 7 d 650 mg t.i.d. P.O. x 7 d
Cryptosporidium parvum	 paromomycin nitazoxanide	self-limited in normal hosts 25 mg/kg/d divided t.i.d. or q.i.d. but duration of therapy is unknown 500 mg (1 tablet or 25 mL suspension▲) q 12 h with food x 3 d
Cyclospora	TMP/SMX	160/800 mg (double-strength tablet) P.O. b.i.d. x 7 d
Cysticercosis***	albendazole or praziquantel	400 mg b.i.d. P.O. x 8 d can use up to 30 days but efficacy not proven 50 mg/kg/q.d. in t.i.d. x 15 d surgery may be alternative treatment
E multilocularis	mebendazole	surgery is treatment of choice followed by medical therapy of prolonged duration with mebendazole 40-50 mg/kg/d in t.i.d. dosing for 2 years after radical surgery or longer for inoperable cysts
Echinococcus (hydatid cyst)	albendazole	400 mg b.i.d. P.O. x 28 d

* For update, see *Med Lett Drugs Ther* 1998;40(1017):1-12.
To get drugs through CDC: 404-639-3670 working hours 8 AM-4:30 PM 404-639-2888; nonbusiness hours, emergencies only.

** Azithromycin and atovaquone may have clinical efficacy, but not FDA approved.

*** An ophthalmic examination should be done before treatment. Corticosteroids should be given for 2-3 d before and during drug therapy for neurocysticercosis.

▲ 10 mL suspension for children 4-11 years of age; tablet form is not for use in children.

Parasite	Drug	Dose (Adult)
Enterobius	pyrantel pamoate mebendazole albendazole	11 mg/kg x 1 dose, repeat after 2 wk 100 mg P.O. x 1 dose, repeat after 2 wk 400 mg P.O. x 1 dose, repeat after 2 wk
Giardia lamblia	metronidazole furazolidone nitazoxanide	250 mg t.i.d. P.O. x 5 d 100 mg q.i.d. P.O. for 7-10 d 500 mg (1 tablet or 25 mL suspension) q 12 h with food x 3 d
Isospora belli	TMP/SMX*	160 mg TMP/800 mg SMX q.i.d. x 10 d then b.i.d. x 3 wk For AIDS patients, add TMP/SMX (160 mg/800 mg) b.i.d. x 10 d
leishmaniasis	sodium stibogluconate**	20 mg/kg/q.d. IV or IM 20-28 d in 2 divided doses
	or meglumine antimonite**	20 mg/kg/q.d. 20-28 d
	or amphotericin B	0.5-1 mg/kg/q.d. or q 2 d up to 8 wk
	or liposomal amphotericin B***	3 mg/kg on days 1-5, then on days 14 and 21
	or amphotericin B colloidal dispersion:	2 mg/kg/d x 10 d
	or amphotericin B lipid complex:	3 mg/kg/d q.o.d. x 5 doses
	or pentamidine	2-4 mg/kg/q.d. or q 2 d IM up to 15 doses
lice†	1% permethrin 1% lindane cream	apply to scalp x 1 dose apply topically x 1 dose

* Investigational for this indication.

** Neither drug licensed for use in United States. CDC has sodium stibogluconate available via compassionate drug use program.

*** AmBisome has been approved by FDA for the treatment of visceral leishmaniasis.

† All topical agents may be reapplied in week if lice still present. Ivermectin 200 µg/kg P.O. x 1 dose investigational for this condition.

continued on next page

Pentamidine Isethionate: An antiprotozoal agent effective against *Pneumocystis jiroveci.* It may inhibit DNA and RNA synthesis. Although little is known of the pharmacology, levels of 0.3 to 0.5 μg/mL have been observed.

The drug has been associated with hypotension, hypoglycemia, and car-

Parasite	Drug	Dose (Adult)
malaria* *Plasmodium falciparum*	chloroquine	Oral therapy: **If chloroquine sensitive:** chloroquine 1 g P.O. followed in 6 h by 500 mg P.O., then 500 mg/d P.O. for 2 more d.
	quinidine gluconate**	IV therapy: **If chloroquine sensitive:** 10 mg/kg loading dose (max 600 mg) in normal saline over 1-2 h; then 0.02 mg/kg/min; change to P.O. if possible;
	or chloroquine	or chloroquine 200 mg IM q 6 h, not to exceed 800 mg the first 24 h
	quinine sulfate	**If chloroquine resistant:** 650 mg q 8 h x 3-7 d plus doxycycline 100 mg q.d. x 7 d, or plus clindamycin 900 mg t.i.d. x 5 d, or pyrimethamine/ sulfadoxine—3 tabs given on last day of quinine therapy
	or mefloquine***	1.25 g x 1 dose, or 750 mg initially followed by 500 mg at 12 h
	or atovaquone	1,000 mg q.d. P.O. x 3 d plus proguanil 400 mg q.d. P.O. x 3 d or plus doxycycline 100 mg b.i.d. P.O. x 3 d
	or quinidine gluconate (IV therapy)	10 mg/kg loading dose (max 600 mg) in normal saline over 1-2 h; then 0.02 mg/kg/min; change to P.O. if possible

* For updated information on malaria treatment and resistance patterns, clinicians should consult the Centers for Disease Control and Prevention in Atlanta, GA: malaria fax hotline: 1-888-232-3299 and/or http://www.cdc.gov/travel/diseases.htm and click on 'malaria'.

** IV quinidine gluconate requires cardiac monitoring (reports of prolonged QT intervals) and glucose monitoring. Loading dose should be omitted in patients who have received P.O. quinine or mefloquine.

*** Neuropsychiatric and cardiac arrhythmias may occur; this drug should not be given to patients with cardiac arrhythmias or to those who are taking drugs that may affect conduction (ie, halofantrine and quinine).
Malarone™ is 250 mg atovaquone and 100 mg proguanil hydrochloride.

diac arrhythmias. There are strict requirements for administration *and the package insert should be used as a guide for therapy*. The usual dose is 4 mg/kg/d for 14 days for *Pneumocystis jiroveci* pneumonitis; for AIDS patients who are seriously ill, 21 days is recommended. Has role as prophylaxis either aerosolized or injectable in AIDS patients.

Parasite	Drug	Dose (Adult)
Plasmodium vivax	chloroquine plus primaquine	1 g, then 500 mg in 6 h, then 500 mg/d x 2 d; then follow by primaquine 15 mg/d x 14 d or
	atovaquone/ proguanil plus primaquine	atovaquone 1,000 mg q.d./ proguanil 400 mg q.d. P.O. x 3 d* followed by primaquine 15 mg/d x 14 d **If chloroquine resistant:** See recommendations for chloroquine-resistant falciparum, followed by primaquine 15 mg/d x 14 d
*Pneumocystis jiroveci***	TMP/SMX	Moderate-severe disease: TMP 15 mg/kg/d x 21 d in oral or IV dosing, t.i.d. or q.i.d.
	pentamidine isethionate	4 mg/kg/d x 21 d
	primaquine plus clindamycin	primaquine 30 mg base q.d. P.O. plus clindamycin 300-600 mg q 6 h P.O., together x 21 d
	trimetrexate glucuronate + leucovorin for injection***	trimetrexate: 45 mg/m²/d x 21 d leucovorin: 20 mg/m² q 6 h x 21 d Indication: alternative therapy for treatment of moderate to severe PCP in immunocompromised patients who are refractory or intolerant to TMP/SMX or for whom it is contraindicated.
	atovaquone or trimethoprim plus dapsone	Mild-moderate disease: 750 mg b.i.d. P.O. x 21 d 5 mg/kg t.i.d. P.O. plus 100 mg q.d. P.O., together x 21 d

* Only if patient did not take this for prophylaxis of malaria.

** For all patients with *P jiroveci* pneumonia, if room air PO_2 <70 mm Hg or A-a gradient >35 mm Hg, should give prednisone 40 mg b.i.d. P.O. x 5 d, then 40 mg q.d. P.O. x 5 d, then 20 mg q.d. x 11 d.

*** See package insert for dosage and toxicities.

continued on next page

Common Parasitic Infections and Treatment *(continued)*

Parasite	Drug	Dose (Adult)
scabies	5% permethrin or 10% crotamiton, or gamma benzene hexachloride	apply topically ivermectin 200 μg/kg x 1 dose (investigational for this condition)
Naegleria	amphotericin B plus rifampin plus ketoconazole	1 mg/kg/d 600 mg/d 200 to 400 mg/d
S mansoni	praziquantel	40 mg/kg/d in 2 doses x 1 d
S haematobium *S japonicum*	praziquantel or oxamniquine	60 mg/kg/d in 2 doses x 1 d or 15 mg/kg/d x 1 dose 20 mg/kg/d x 3 d in North and East Africa 30 mg/kg/d x 2 d in Egypt and South Africa
Strongyloides	ivermectin thiabendazole* albendazole	200 μg/kg/d P.O. x 1-2 d 50 mg/kg/d in 2 doses (max 3 g/d) 400 mg q.d. P.O. x 3 d
Tapeworm infections: *Taenia solium* (pork tapeworm) *Taenia saginatum* (beef tapeworm) *Taenia diphyllobothrium latum* (fish tapeworm)	albendazole praziquantel niclosamide	15 mg/kg/d b.i.d. (max 400 mg b.i.d.) x 8-30 d 50 mg/kg/d t.i.d. x 30 d Four 500-mg chewable tablets x 1 d

*For disseminated disease, treat with thiabendazole for 7 d.

Parasite	Drug	Dose (Adult)
Toxoplasma gondii	pyrimethamine plus sulfadiazine leucovorin	25-100 mg/d x 3-4 wk plus 1-1.5 g q.i.d. x 3-4 wk plus 10 mg q.d. P.O. with each dose of pyrimethamine
		Cerebral toxoplasmosis in AIDS:
	pyrimethamine	200 mg P.O. x 1 then, 75-100 mg q.d. P.O. plus
	sulfadiazine	1-1.5 g q.i.d. P.O. plus
	leucovorin	10 mg q.d. P.O. with each dose of pyrimethamine. Can substitute clindamycin 600 mg q 6 h P.O. or IV, sulfa allergic. Treat for 3-6 wk, then patients need lifetime suppression with
	sulfadiazine	500 mg-1,000 mg q.i.d. P.O. plus
	pyrimethamine	25-50 mg q.d. P.O.
	leucovorin	10-25 mg q.d. P.O.
	TMP/SMX	For prophylaxis: TMP/SMX-DS P.O. 1 g q.d. For therapy: TMP/SMX 10-50 mg/kg/d P.O. or IV in 2 divided doses x 30 d
Trichuris trichiura (whipworm)	mebendazole	100 mg b.i.d. P.O. x 3 d or 500 mg P.O. x 1
	albendazole	400 mg P.O. x 1 dose (3 d for heavy infection)
visceral larva migrans (Toxocariasis)	diethylcarbamazine	6 mg/kg t.i.d. x 7-10 d (needs to be obtained via CDC)
	albendazole	400 mg b.i.d. P.O. x 5 d
	mebendazole	100 mg-200 mg b.i.d. P.O. x 5 d
Trypanosoma cruzi	benznidazole	5 mg/kg/day b.i.d. for 60 days
	nifurtimox	10 mg/kg/day either t.i.d. or q.i.d. x 120 days

Section 2: Therapy by Pathogen

Key

— = gram-negative	C = coccus	F = filamentous
+ = gram-positive	C-B = coccobacillary	S = spiral
R = rod or bacillus	A = acid-fast	B = bacillary

Pathogen	Type	Empiric Choices	Supplemental Therapy Needed	Alternatives
Acinetobacter	—, R	piperacillin piperacillin/ tazobactam aminoglycoside TMP/SMX imipenem meropenem		ceftazidime cefepime quinolones ampicillin/ sulbactam (for resistant strains)
Actinobacillus actinomycetem-comitans	—, C-B	amoxicillin	amino-glycoside	
Actinomyces	+, R	penicillin G		clindamycin tetracycline
Aeromonas hydrophila	—, R	aminoglycoside quinolones		TMP/SMX
Bacillary angiomatosis (due to *B henselae* and *B quintana*)		erythromycin or doxycycline		azithromycin clarithromycin
Bacillus anthracis (anthrax)	+, R	ciprofloxacin doxycycline or *penicillin (if sensitive)		possibly other quinolones

*For prophylaxis only.

Pathogen	Type	Empiric Choices	Supplemental Therapy Needed	Alternatives
Bacteroides fragilis	—, R	clindamycin or metronidazole ampicillin/sulbactam piperacillin/ tazobactam imipenem/cilastatin meropenem ertapenem		mezlocillin cefoxitin cefotetan* chloramphenicol amoxicillin/ clavulanate ticarcillin/ clavulanate trovafloxacin**
Bacteroides melanino-genicus	—, R	penicillin G clindamycin cefoxitin cefotetan metronidazole if β-lactamase producer ampicillin/sulbactam piperacillin/ tazobactam		piperacillin mezlocillin tetracycline amoxicillin/ clavulanate ticarcillin/ clavulanate carbapenems
Bartonella henselae (cat scratch, endocarditis)	—, R	azithromycin erythromycin doxycycline clarithromycin quinolone		TMP/SMX doxycycline + rifampin
Bartonella quintana (trench fever)		doxycycline erythromycin		TMP/SMX

* Many strains of *B distasonis*, *B ovatus*, and *B thetaiotaomicron* are resistant in vitro, but this may not predict response.

** Serious to fatal liver damage has occurred, so safer alternative antimicrobial therapy is recommended, when available.

continued on next page

Therapy by Pathogen *(continued)*

Pathogen	Type	Empiric Choices	Supplemental Therapy Needed	Alternatives
Bordetella	—, C-B	erythromycin		TMP/SMX
Borrelia	S	tetracycline		chloramphenicol
Borrelia burgdorferi	S	early diagnosis: cefuroxime doxycycline* erythromycin amoxicillin with/without probenecid late diagnosis: IV penicillin ceftriaxone (neurologic involvement, arthritis)		if allergic to penicillin or tetracycline, then erythromycin could be used; cefuroxime axetil has been used
Brucella	—, R	doxycycline	streptomycin or gentamicin	TMP/SMX
Burkholderia cepacia	—, R	TMP/SMX ciprofloxacin imipenem meropenem ceftazidime		chloramphenicol IV minocycline
Calymmatobacterium granulomatis	—, C-B	doxycycline TMP/SMX		ciprofloxacin azithromycin erythromycin
Campylobacter	—, R	erythromycin		clindamycin doxycycline azithromycin clarithromycin

*Not to be used in pregnant or lactating women or in children under 8 years old.

Pathogen	Type	Empiric Choices	Supplemental Therapy Needed	Alternatives
Capnocytophaga sp	—, R	clindamycin amoxicillin/ clavulanate		ciprofloxacin penicillin G imipenem cefoxitin
Chlamydophila, Chlamydia (*C pneumoniae*)		doxycycline moxifloxacin levofloxacin erythromycin gatifloxacin telithromycin		azithromycin clarithromycin
Chlamydia trachomatis		doxycycline azithromycin		erythromycin succinate levofloxacin ofloxacin
Chromobacterium violaceum	—, R	chloramphenicol		ciprofloxacin imipenem
Citrobacter diversus	—, R	imipenem meropenem ertapenem aztreonam ciprofloxacin levofloxacin		piperacillin mezlocillin piperacillin/ tazobactam 3rd-generation cephalosporins
Citrobacter freundii	—, R	aminoglycosides, quinolones cefepime		piperacillin/ tazobactam
Clostridium botulinum	+, R	antitoxin β-lactam if wound present		
Clostridium difficile	+, R	vancomycin or metronidazole* P.O.	stop antibiotics	cholestyramine

*Poor responses have been reported recently.

continued on next page

Therapy by Pathogen *(continued)*

Pathogen	Type	Empiric Choices	Supplemental Therapy Needed	Alternatives
Clostridium perfringens	+, R	penicillin G metronidazole		clindamycin doxycycline chloramphen-icol IV cefoxitin cefotetan piperacillin/ tazobactam
Clostridium tetani	+, R	penicillin metronidazole	immunization antitoxin	imipenem meropenem
Corynebacterium diphtheriae	+, R	erythromycin		clindamycin penicillin
Corynebacterium diphtheriae, carrier	+, R	erythromycin		
E coli (hospital-acquired)	—, R	ciprofloxacin levofloxacin aminoglycoside aztreonam or cephalosporin piperacillin/ tazobactam carbapenems trovafloxacin*		ampicillin (if sensitive) ticarcillin/ clavulanate piperacillin
E coli (urinary)	—, R	ampicillin** TMP/SMX** quinolone		

* Serious to fatal liver damage has occurred, so safer alternative antimicrobial therapy is recommended, when available.

** Resistant strains are increasing.

Pathogen	Type	Empiric Choices	Supplemental Therapy Needed	Alternatives
Eikenella corrodens	—, R	penicillin G amoxicillin/ clavulanate TMP/SMX quinolone ampicillin		doxycycline cefoxitin cefuroxime imipenem
Enterobacter	—, R	imipenem meropenem cefepime piperacillin/ tazobactam aminoglycoside aztreonam ciprofloxacin		TMP/SMX ticarcillin/ clavulanate* 3rd-generation cephalosporin levofloxacin trovafloxacin**
*Enterococcus faecalis****	+, C	ampicillin or penicillin G	aminoglycoside for treatment of endocarditis or nonresponsive infections	vancomycin piperacillin ampicillin/ sulbactam piperacillin/ tazobactam linezolid
Enterococcus faecium† (VRE)		quinupristin/ dalfopristin linezolid		doxycycline if sensitive for vancomycin-resistant strains of *E faecium* daptomycin (not FDA approved)

* Urinary tract infections only.

** Serious to fatal liver damage has occurred, so safer alternative antimicrobial therapy is recommended, when available.

*** β-lactamase-producing and high-level gentamicin-resistant strains are appearing.

† Multiresistant strains are increasing.

continued on next page

Therapy by Pathogen *(continued)*

Pathogen	Type	Empiric Choices	Supplemental Therapy Needed	Alternatives
Erysipelothrix rhusiopathiae	+, R	penicillin G ampicillin		3rd-generation cephalosporin
Eubacteria	+, R	penicillin		clindamycin tetracycline cefoxitin carbapenems
Flavobacteria	—, R	aminoglycoside 3rd-generation cephalosporin		piperacillin/ tazobactam
Francisella tularensis	—, C-B	gentamicin tobramycin doxycycline ciprofloxacin streptomycin		chloramphenicol IV
Fusobacteria	—, R	penicillin G clindamycin		cefoxitin piperacillin/ tazobactam
Gardnerella vaginalis	—, R	metronidazole	clindamycin	
Haemophilus aphrophilus	—, R	cephalothin ampicillin ampicillin/ sulbactam	aminoglycoside	piperacillin quinolones 2nd- or 3rd-generation cephalosporins

Pathogen	Type	Empiric Choices	Supplemental Therapy Needed	Alternatives
Haemophilus influenzae	—, R, C, B	ampicillin moxifloxacin ciprofloxacin gatifloxacin azithromycin telithromycin cefuroxime amoxicillin/clav. ticarcillin/clav. ceftibuten 2nd-, 3rd-, or 4th-generation cephalosporins TMP/SMX aztreonam ofloxacin levofloxacin piperacillin/ tazobactam cefixime		chloramphenicol IV (possibly in meningitis) trovafloxacin* cefditoren clarithromycin
Haemophilus ducreyi	—, R	erythromycin azithromycin ceftriaxone ciprofloxacin	if resistant in vitro, test to sensitivity rifampin cefoxitin	minocycline
Haemophilus parainfluenzae	—, R	ampicillin ciprofloxacin moxifloxacin gatifloxacin trovafloxacin*		ceftibuten cefdinir chloramphenicol TMP/SMX

*Serious to fatal liver damage has occurred, so safer alternative antimicrobial therapy is recommended, when available.

continued on next page

Therapy by Pathogen *(continued)*

Pathogen	Type	Empiric Choices	Supplemental Therapy Needed	Alternatives
Helicobacter pylori	—, R	clarithromycin plus either: • omeprazole, or • ranitidine + bismuth citrate		
JK-Diphtheroids	+, R	vancomycin		erythromycin
Kingella kingae	—, C-B	cephalosporins penicillin		rifampin*
Klebsiella pneumoniae	—, R	imipenem/cilastatin meropenem ertapenem ciprofloxacin ofloxacin cefepime piperacillin/tazobactam 3rd-generation cephalosporins	aminoglycoside aztreonam	piperacillin mezlocillin ticarcillin/clavulanate trovafloxacin**
Lactobacillus confusus	+, C	penicillin G ampicillin	gentamicin	resistant to vancomycin clindamycin erythromycin
Legionella sp *Legionella pneumophila*	R	erythromycin dirithromycin azithromycin*** gatifloxacin trovafloxacin**	rifampin	clarithromycin† telithromycin†
Leptospira	—,S	penicillin		doxycycline

*Used as prophylaxis.

**Serious to fatal liver damage has occurred, so safer alternative antimicrobial therapy is recommended, when available.

***In vitro sensitivities; not FDA approved for oral agent; approved for IV only.

†In vitro only; not FDA approved.

Pathogen	Type	Empiric Choices	Supplemental Therapy Needed	Alternatives
Leuconostoc mesenteroides	+, C	minocycline* penicillin G ampicillin clindamycin erythromycin		resistant to vancomycin
Listeria monocytogenes	+, R	ampicillin TMP/SMX	aminoglycoside	erythromycin penicillin G (high-dose)
Moraxella catarrhalis	—, C	amoxicillin/clavulanate (including XR) moxifloxacin TMP/SMX ciprofloxacin clarithromycin azithromycin telithromycin loracarbef ceftibuten cefpodoxime proxetil gatifloxacin cefixime cefuroxime axetil cefprozil cefdinir levofloxacin ofloxacin		cefaclor dirithromycin erythromycin doxycycline cefditoren
Morganella morganii	—, R	imipenem meropenem cefotaxime cefepime ciprofloxacin levofloxacin ertapenem		aminoglycoside piperacillin/tazobactam aztreonam

*These are in vitro sensitivities only.

continued on next page

Therapy by Pathogen *(continued)*

Pathogen	Type	Empiric Choices	Supplemental Therapy Needed	Alternatives
mycobacteria, nontuberculous 'atypical'* 1) slow growers: *M avium-intracellulare* complex	Acid-fast rods ↓	clarithromycin** or azithromycin + ethambutol + rifabutin (some/all)	surgery	amikacin rifampin
M scrofulaceum		as above	surgery	
M kansasii		isoniazid + ethambutol + streptomycin or isoniazid + ethambutol + rifampin		clarithromycin ethionamide
M marinum		minocycline doxycycline	surgery	TMP/SMX rifampin + ethambutol clarithromycin
M xenopi		isoniazid + streptomycin + rifampin		
2) rapid growers: *M fortuitum*	May resemble diphtheroids on Gram stain ↓	amikacin + cefoxitin		TMP/SMX ethambutol doxycycline
M chelonae		clarithromycin ± amikacin or imipenem		
M leprae		rifampin + dapsone, and, if needed, clofazimine		quinolones clarithromycin minocycline

* After empiric therapy, it is necessary to treat on the basis of antibiotic sensitivity.
** See package insert for dosing information.

Pathogen	Type	Empiric Choices	Supplemental Therapy Needed	Alternatives
Mycoplasma pneumoniae		erythromycin clarithromycin azithromycin telithromycin moxifloxacin levofloxacin gatifloxacin dirithromycin trovafloxacin*		minocycline (not in children) doxycycline (not in children)
Neisseria gonorrhoeae	—, C	ceftriaxone cefixime ciprofloxacin levofloxacin		
PPNG		ceftriaxone cefuroxime cefotaxime spectinomycin TMP/SMX levofloxacin cefpodoxime proxetil gatifloxacin		piperacillin/ tazobactam
Neisseria meningitidis	—, C	penicillin G ampicillin		chloramphenicol cefuroxime 3rd- or 4th-generation cephalosporin, ciprofloxacin as prophylaxis
Nocardia asteroides	+, R, A, F	TMP/SMX		minocycline + amikacin carbapenems

* Serious to fatal liver damage has occurred, so safer alternative antimicrobial therapy is recommended, when available.

continued on next page

Therapy by Pathogen *(continued)*

Pathogen	Type	Empiric Choices	Supplemental Therapy Needed	Alternatives
Pasteurella multocida	—, R	penicillin G cefuroxime axetil ampicillin amoxicillin		TMP/SMX amoxicillin/clav. loracarbef doxycycline
Peptococcus	+, C	penicillin G		clindamycin cefotetan cefoxitin tetracycline amoxicillin/clavulanate ticarcillin/clavulanate piperacillin piperacillin/tazobactam
Peptostreptococcus	+, C	penicillin G clindamycin		cefotetan cefoxitin amoxicillin/clavulanate ticarcillin/clavulanate piperacillin piperacillin/tazobactam erythromycin doxycycline vancomycin carbapenems trovafloxacin*
Propionibacterium acnes	+, R	tetracycline		clindamycin (topical) minocycline
Proteus (indole-positive)	—, R	3rd- or 4th-generation cephalosporin aminoglycoside ciprofloxacin ofloxacin ticarcillin/clavulanate piperacillin/tazobactam		cefoxitin piperacillin ertapenem imipenem meropenem

* Serious to fatal liver damage has occurred, so safer alternative antimicrobial therapy is recommended, when available.

Pathogen	Type	Empiric Choices	Supplemental Therapy Needed	Alternatives
Proteus mirabilis	—, R	TMP/SMX ampicillin cephalosporin ciprofloxacin ofloxacin piperacillin/tazobactam		trovafloxacin*
Providencia	—, R	TMP/SMX 3rd-generation cephalosporin aztreonam amikacin ciprofloxacin ofloxacin levofloxacin		cefoxitin cefotetan piperacillin ticarcillin piperacillin/ tazobactam
Pseudo-monas aeruginosa	—, R	ceftazidime cefepime tobramycin or gentamicin or aztreonam + piperacillin or ticarcillin/clavulanate, or piperacillin/tazobactam;** ciprofloxacin*** cefoperazone imipenem meropenem		
Rickettsia	—, C-B	doxycycline		quinolones chloramphenicol IV
Salmonella	—, R	ceftriaxone ciprofloxacin ofloxacin amoxicillin		TMP/SMX
Salmonella typhi	—, R	ceftriaxone amoxicillin ciprofloxacin ofloxacin		chloramphenicol IV TMP/SMX

* Serious to fatal liver damage has occurred, so safer alternative antimicrobial therapy is recommended, when available.

** An aminoglycoside should be added.

*** Most active quinolone, active orally and IV.

continued on next page

Therapy by Pathogen *(continued)*

Pathogen	Type	Empiric Choices	Supplemental Therapy Needed	Alternatives
Serratia	—, R	3rd-generation cephalosporin or aztreonam or piperacillin + aminoglycoside ciprofloxacin cefepime ertapenem imipenem meropenem		levofloxacin piperacillin/ tazobactam
Shigella	—, R	ciprofloxacin ofloxacin		ampicillin TMP/SMX
Spirillum	—, R	penicillin		tetracycline
Staphylococcus aureus (penicillinase-producing)	+, C	nafcillin/ oxacillin cefazolin	aminoglycoside may be synergistic; useful early in serious infections?	vancomycin moxifloxacin cefepime clarithromycin* azithromycin* telithromycin** cefdinir amoxicillin/clav. ticarcillin/clav. piperacillin/ tazobactam quinupristin/ dalfopristin loracarbef* dirithromycin* carbapenems

* For uncomplicated skin infections only. Approved in IV for community-acquired pneumonia. Oral agent approved for skin and skin structure infections.

** Methicillin- and erythromycin-sensitive only.

Pathogen	Type	Empiric Choices	Supplemental Therapy Needed	Alternatives
Staphylococcus aureus (methicillin-resistant)	+, C	vancomycin linezolid daptomycin quinupristin/dalfopristin*	rifampin (?)	TMP/SMX has been successful in some cases.* Tetracycline, clindamycin, and TMP/SMX may be active against community-acquired MRSA strains.
Staphylococcus epidermidis	+, C	nafcillin** or oxacillin**	vancomycin	
Staphylococcus epidermidis (methicillin-resistant)	+, C	vancomycin	rifampin or gentamicin	linezolid
Stentotrophomonas maltophilia	—, R	TMP/SMX		aztreonam ticarcillin/clavulanate minocycline doxycycline
Streptobacillus moniliformis	—, R	penicillin doxycycline		erythromycin clindamycin

*Not released for this indication.

**If sensitive and not on prosthetic device; otherwise use vancomycin.

continued on next page

Therapy by Pathogen *(continued)*

Pathogen	Type	Empiric Choices	Supplemental Therapy Needed	Alternatives
Streptococcus agalactiae (group B)	+, C	penicillin G	aminoglycoside (often)	erythromycin trovafloxacin* azithromycin carbapenems
Streptococcus bovis (D)	+, C	penicillin G		cephalosporin clindamycin
*Streptococcus pneumoniae***	+, C	penicillin G ceftriaxone levofloxacin moxifloxacin gatifloxacin azithromycin vancomycin*** amoxicillin/ clavulanate XR▲ cephalosporins respiratory telithromycin† amoxicillin	rifampin	erythromycin clindamycin clarithromycin dirithromycin cefepime cefdinir cefpodoxime proxetil loracarbef ticarcillin/clav. piperacillin/ tazobactam linezolid carbapenems cefditoren

* Serious to fatal liver damage has occurred, so safer alternative antimicrobial therapy is recommended, when available.

** Multiresistant strains are increasing.

*** Penicillin-resistant strains have been reported in United States. The drugs of choice for these strains are respiratory quinolones, or third-generation cephalosporins, or vancomycin plus ceftriaxone or cefotaxime, plus rifampin for meningitis.

▲ FDA approved for strains with reduced susceptibility to PCN with MICs of 2 μg/mL.

† Including multidrug-resistant strains in community-acquired pneumonia.

Pathogen	Type	Empiric Choices	Supplemental Therapy Needed	Alternatives
Streptococcus pyogenes (A)	+, C	penicillin		erythromycin cefdinir cephalosporin clindamycin amoxicillin/clav. clarithromycin azithromycin cefpodoxime proxetil loracarbef dirithromycin* piperacillin/tazobactam quinupristin/dalfopristin linezolid ticarcillin/clav. carbapenems
Streptococcus viridans	+, C	penicillin G	gentamicin (may be necessary in some cases)	cephalosporin vancomycin clindamycin
Treponema pallidum	—, S	penicillin G		erythromycin doxycycline tetracycline
Ureaplasma urealyticum		tetracyclines		erythromycin levofloxacin
Vibrio cholerae	—, R	fluids + doxycycline		quinolones TMP/SMX
Vibrio vulnificus	—, R	doxycycline quinolones		TMP/SMX
Yersinia enterocolitica	—, R	aminoglycoside TMP/SMX		quinolones
Yersinia pestis	—, R	streptomycin gentamicin	tetracycline	chloramphenicol doxycycline ciprofloxacin

*Effective for pharyngitis.

continued on next page

Therapy by Pathogen *(continued)*

Pathogen	Type	Empiric Choices	Supplemental Therapy Needed	Alternatives
Fungi				
Aspergillus sp		voriconazole amphotericin B (including lipid preparations)	tetracycline has been added to other antifungals	5-flucytosine (used successfully in some pulmonary cases) itraconazole* caspofungin*
Blastomyces dermatitidis		amphotericin B		itraconazole
Candida sp		fluconazole amphotericin B (including lipid preparations) caspofungin voriconazole		5-flucytosine (use with other agents) itraconazole micafungin**
Coccidioides immitis		amphotericin B		ketoconazole itraconazole*** fluconazole***
Cryptococcus neoformans		amphotericin B	5-flucytosine	fluconazole itraconazole***
Chromoblastomyces		itraconazole 5-flucytosine ketoconazole	terbinafine	amphotericin B

* FDA approved for this indication in patients refractory or intolerant to amphotericin B therapy.

** Only approved for esophageal candidiasis and prophylaxis in stem-cell transplant patients.

*** Not FDA approved for this indication.

Pathogen	Type	Empiric Choices	Supplemental Therapy Needed	Alternatives
dermatophytes		clotrimazole		fluconazole* itraconazole voriconazole
Fusarium		amphotericin B voriconazole	rifampin	
Histoplasma		amphotericin B		itraconazole fluconazole*
mucormycosis zygomycosis		Lipid preparations ABLC or LAMB amphotericin B		posaconazole**
Paracoccidioides		itraconazole ketoconazole	amphotericin B	
Penicillium		amphotericin B		itraconazole
Sporotrichum		iodide itraconazole		itraconazole* amphotericin B
Phialophora (chromomycosis)		itraconazole		
Pseudallescheria boydii		voriconazole		
Scedosporium		voriconazole		

*Not FDA approved for this indication.
**Experimental and only available orally.

Section 3: Ear, Nose, and Throat Infections

George A. Pankey, MD

Sinusitis is one of the most common health-care complaints in the United States, affecting approximately 1 in 8 persons at some time in their lives. An estimated 37 million Americans are affected by sinusitis each year. This estimate suggests that sinusitis is diagnosed more frequently than hypertension, arthritis, and all other adult respiratory diseases. It has become the number one chronic illness for all age groups in the United States, according to the National Center for Disease Statistics. Sinusitis was the most commonly reported chronic disease, affecting an estimated 14% of the population in the United States.

Most patients with sinusitis are treated medically by primary care physicians, although increasing numbers of patients with recurrent and chronic sinusitis are being treated surgically. In fact, some estimates indicate that more than 200,000 sinus surgical procedures are being performed each year in the United States. The number of patients treated surgically could decline if primary care physicians took a more aggressive medical management approach. Therefore, it is important for primary care physicians to recognize and properly diagnose acute, chronic, and acute exacerbations of chronic sinusitis, even though identifying the causes of recurrent and chronic sinusitis can be challenging. Treatment should be aimed at eliminating causative factors and controlling the inflammatory as well as the infectious components of the disease.

Antimicrobial therapy is useful in the management of sinusitis when used in conjunction with relief of obstruction and with other appropriate therapy. The purpose of therapy for presumed bacterial sinusitis is to return the sinuses to normal, to avoid development of chronic sinusitis, and to prevent respiratory, orbital, and intracranial complications.

The emergence of penicillin-resistant bacterial sinus pathogens has rendered amoxicillin and trimethoprim/sulfamethoxazole less useful in many parts of the United States.

No antimicrobial agent has been approved for use in *chronic* sinusitis or acute exacerbations of chronic sinusitis; however, the choice of antibiotic for acute exacerbations is no different than that for acute sinusitis. If there is any sign of maxillary dental problems, suspicion of anaerobes rises in the patient with chronic sinusitis, making an agent with antianaerobic activity preferable.

Pseudomonas aeruginosa, staphylococci, and anaerobes are more commonly isolated from patients with chronic vs acute sinusitis.

Knowledge of the antimicrobial susceptibility pattern of the organisms most likely to be associated with community-acquired sinusitis in your geographic area is necessary in choosing empiric therapy. Because β-lactamase-producing strains of *H influenzae* and *M catarrhalis* are common in most areas of the United States, ampicillin, amoxicillin, cefuroxime axetil, cefpodoxime, and loracarbef would not be first-choice agents. If the clinician is concerned about penicillin-resistant *S pneumoniae*, gatifloxacin, levofloxacin, and moxifloxacin are better choices for the outpatient with sinusitis. If sinusitis is associated with maxillary dental disease, anaerobes are more likely to be involved, and amoxicillin/clavulanic acid, doxycycline, or moxifloxacin would be good choices for oral therapy.

Adherence to treatment for any infectious disease is important. It maximizes the chances that the treatment will be efficacious and minimizes the possibility of bacterial resistance. Shorter course therapies have been shown to enhance adherence. Examples include a single-dose for azithromycin or once-daily dosing for cefdinir, gatifloxacin, levofloxacin, moxifloxacin, and telithromycin. Azithromycin now also comes in a single, 2-g oral suspension dose. Telithromycin was the first ketolide approved by the FDA for the treatment of acute bacterial sinusitis. This is a new drug in the macrolide family. The dosage regimen for telithromycin is one tablet each day for 5 days. Amoxicillin/clavulanate, cefpodoxime, cefprozil, cefuroxime axetil, ciprofloxacin, clarithromycin, doxycycline, and loracarbef are given twice daily.

Patients who fail to respond to initial antimicrobial therapy for bacterial sinusitis should have a limited computed tomography (CT) scan taken of the sinuses. A consultation should be made with an otolaryngologist. This specialist usually will perform an endoscopic evaluation and obtain a specimen for culture and sensitivity. If the CT scan shows no fluid accumulation that would require surgical drainage, a change of antibiotic should be considered.

Important Considerations

- Viral rhinosinusitis is common and cannot be clinically distinguished from bacterial sinusitis for 7 days.
- Viral rhinosinusitis responds to placebo just as well as to antibacterials (ie, it is self-limiting).
- Antimicrobials may be beneficial to patients with viral rhinosinusitis whose nasopharyngeal secretions contain *H influenzae, M catarrhalis, or S pneumoniae.*
- If a patient is still ill after 1 week of presumed viral rhinosinusitis, antimicrobial therapy plus a decongestant are beneficial.
- The appropriate length of antimicrobial therapy has not been established for acute sinusitis. FDA-approved therapeutic regimens are single dose (azithromycin extended release), 3 days (azithromycin), 5 days (levofloxacin, telithromycin), or 10 days (10 other FDA-approved antibacterials) of therapy. Longer therapy (21 days or more) is frequently used for patients with acute exacerbations of chronic sinusitis, but without supporting data.
- The agents effective for acute sinusitis are also effective for acute exacerbations of chronic sinusitis; however, the prevalence of anaerobic bacteria in the latter is increased.

Ear, Nose, and Throat Infections *(continued)*

External otitis (infective)

Eczematoid dermatitis, furuncle, reaction to foreign object. Itching, pain, dryness. Discharge, decreased hearing. Adenopathy, fever.

Otitis Media

Onset post-URI, fever, pain. Dullness and hyperemia of tympanum-bulging.

Mastoiditis

Complication of otitis media. Mastoid tenderness, fever, pain, x-ray bone destruction.

Chronic mastoiditis usually requires surgery in addition to antibiotics.

Sinusitis

History of URI. Pain, tenderness, nasal congestion, and purulent nasal discharge. Fever, chills, malaise, headache, and maxillary dental pain.

Acute Tonsillitis

Sore throat, fever, inflamed tonsils with exudate. Cervical lymphadenopathy. Leukocytosis. Differential diagnosis: group A streptococci, herpes simplex, and infectious mononucleosis.

Location	Primary Diagnosis	Secondary Diagnosis/ Contributing Factors	Pathogens
Ear	otitis externa	swimmer's ear	*Pseudomonas* sp coliforms *S aureus* (acute)
		furuncle	*S aureus*
		furuncle + cellulitis	*S aureus*
		chronic	generally associated with seborrhea
		malignant external otitis	*Pseudomonas aeruginosa*

Chronic Pharyngitis

Although exact etiology uncertain, chronic Epstein-Barr virus (EBV) infections are associated clinically.

Chronic Tonsillitis

After repeated tonsillitis. Persistent hyperemia, edema of tonsils, fetid breath. Tonsillar size unimportant. Treatment: surgery may be necessary.

Peritonsillar Abscess

After tonsillitis. Unilateral sore throat, dysphagia, unilateral displacement of uvula fluctuant mass. *Drainage necessary* in addition to antibiotics.

Acute Laryngitis

After rhinitis, pharyngitis, influenza, measles, etc. Hoarseness, pain, cough, stridor, red mucosa, exudate, occasional slight hemoptysis. Viral etiology usual.

3

Empiric Choices	Alternatives	Duration	Other Measures/ Comments
polymyxin B + neomycin + hydrocortisone drops	ciprofloxacin HC drops	as needed	Dry after swimming. No ointments.
incision and drainage	if clinical condition warrants, add antibiotics		Antibiotics as ancillary measures, if indicated.
dicloxacillin TMP/SMX	cephalexin, clindamycin	7-10 d	Incision and drainage.
polymyxin B + neomycin + hydrocortisone drops	eardrops: polymyxin + neomycin + hydrocortisone ciprofloxacin HC otic	as needed	Treat seborrhea.
piperacillin, ceftazidime ciprofloxacin ± tobramycin	cefepime	6-12 wk	Surgical drainage, mastoidectomy, regulation of diabetes. Ciprofloxacin HC drops.

continued on next page

Location	Primary Diagnosis	Secondary Diagnosis/ Contributing Factors	Pathogens
Ear *(continued)*	otitis media	neonatal	*S pneumoniae* *H influenzae*, coliforms (*E coli, Klebsiella*), group A and B streptococci
		children	*Pneumococcus* *H influenzae* group A streptococci *M catarrhalis*
	mastoiditis	acute	*Pneumococcus* *H influenzae* group A streptococci
		chronic	coliforms *Pseudomonas* mixed anaerobes *S aureus*

Empiric Choices	Alternatives	Duration	Other Measures/ Comments
ceftriaxone plus vancomycin		10 d	Perform tympanocentesis. Prescribe according to smear. Alter with culture result. Check hearing later.
amoxicillin (if no antibiotic in previous month)	cefuroxime axetil amoxicillin/clav. cefixime cefaclor TMP/SMX cefdinir cefprozil clarithromycin azithromycin cefpodoxime proxetil loracarbef* ceftibuten	1-14 d	Nontypable. *H influenzae* resistant to amoxicillin—in some areas more than 30% β-lactamase resistance reported. The alternative agents are effective vs β-lactamase-producing *H influenzae, M catarrhalis.*
ceftriaxone	moxifloxacin	14-21 d	Antibiotic adjustment based on culture from surgery.
piperacillin/ tazobactam	moxifloxacin	4-6 wk	Antibiotic adjustment based on culture from surgery.

*In a patient population with significant numbers of β-lactamase-producing organisms, cure and bacteriologic eradication rates were somewhat less than those observed with a product containing a β-lactamase inhibitor.

continued on next page

Ear, Nose, and Throat Infections *(continued)*

Location	Primary Diagnosis	Secondary Diagnosis/ Contributing Factors	Pathogens
Pharynx	exudative pharyngitis	tonsillitis	group A streptococci
	diphtheria	membranous pharyngitis	*C diphtheriae*
	epiglottiditis		*H influenzae*
	Vincent's infection	necrotizing pharyngitis	spirochetes anaerobes
	peritonsillar abscess		*S aureus* anaerobes *S pyogenes*

Empiric Choices	Alternatives	Duration	Other Measures/ Comments
benzathine penicillin G penicillin V	amoxicillin amoxicillin/ clavulanate cefpodoxime proxetil clindamycin loracarbef clarithromycin azithromycin cefdinir cefditoren	5*-10** d	Culture and fluorescent antibody type. Consider mononucleosis.
erythromycin to decrease carrier state	benzathine penicillin G penicillin V	10 d	Antitoxin to treat disease. Tracheostomy if needed. Isolation until cultures negative.
cefuroxime cefotaxime ceftriaxone	ampicillin/ sulbactam IV levofloxacin moxifloxacin gatifloxacin	10 d	Primary drug based on knowledge of bacteria sensitivities of environment.
penicillin or clindamycin	cefoxitin piperacillin/ tazobactam doxycycline	10 d	Gram stain reveals fusiform bacteria, spirochetes. Some *Bacteroides* strains produce β-lactamase, inactivating penicillin.
nafcillin or oxacillin or if MRSA, vancomycin + cefoxitin or clindamycin	ticarcillin/ clavulanate piperacillin/ tazobactam	10 d	X-ray; surgery usually.

*Azithromycin
**Penicillin G and penicillin V must be 10 days.

continued on next page

3

Location	Primary Diagnosis	Secondary Diagnosis/ Contributing Factors	Pathogens
Sinuses (paranasal)	acute bacterial sinusitis	acute	*Pneumococcus** *H influenzae* *M catarrhalis* group A streptococci *S aureus* (less frequent)
		chronic	polymicrobic including anaerobes

* Bacterial diagnosis should be established only by sinus aspiration.

Empiric Choices	Alternatives	Duration	Other Measures/ Comments
amoxicillin amoxicillin/ clavulanate azithromycin* cefdinir cefprozil cefuroxime axetil** clarithromycin doxycycline*** gatifloxacin*** levofloxacin*** moxifloxacin*** telithromycin	cefixime cefaclor cefpodoxime proxetil vancomycin IV + ceftriaxone IV for severe infections	Depending on agent, length of therapy varies from 1-10 d.	Drainage, decongestants. Use parenteral drugs, ie, ceftriaxone, if patient is seriously ill.
amoxicillin/ clavulanate moxifloxacin***	doxycycline*** clindamycin	14-21 d	Surgery often necessary.

* Available in 500-mg tablets for 3 days, and in single-dose extended release 2 g for oral suspension.

** Indicated for *S pneumoniae* and for non-β-lactamase-producing strains of *H influenzae*. Insufficient numbers of isolates of β-lactamase-producing strains of *H influenzae* and *M catarrhalis* were obtained from clinical trials with cefuroxime axetil for patients with acute bacterial maxillary sinusitis.

***Not approved for use in children.

Section 4: Respiratory Tract Infections

Antonio Anzueto, MD

Acute Exacerbations of Chronic Bronchitis (AECB)

Despite the controversy over the need to prescribe antibiotics for patients with AECB, high-risk patients have been identified who will benefit from this therapy. These include patients with a history of repeated infections (>4 per year), with comorbid illnesses (such as diabetes, asthma, coronary heart disease), or with marked airway obstruction.

Many of the earlier clinical studies showed either no benefit, or minimal benefit, when antibiotics were prescribed, but these results were mainly due to the study design and the patient population studied. A more recent, larger, international, multicenter, randomized, double-blind study (MOSAIC) compared the effectiveness of oral moxifloxacin 400 mg once daily with standard oral 7-day antibiotic treatment regimens (amoxicillin, cefuroxime, and clarithromycin) as a first-line therapy for infectious AECB. This study demonstrated that moxifloxacin was equivalent to the comparator regimen for the primary outcome (ie, clinical success at 7 to 10 days post-therapy). Superiority with moxifloxacin was shown for both short- and long-term efficacy variables, including cure rate, need for additional antimicrobial treatment, rate of bacteriologic eradication, and time to next exacerbation. Benefits appear to be evident for all subgroups of patients but especially greater in patients with more frequent exacerbations in prior years and in those not receiving systemic steroids. (Wilson et al, *Chest* 2004;125:953-964.)

Community-Acquired Pneumonia

For ambulatory patients, the FDA has recently approved the following treatment regimens:

- Azithromycin extended-release oral suspension single dose 2 g was as effective as 5 to 7 days of treatment with extended-release clarithromycin or levofloxacin.
- High-dose fluoroquinolones, levofloxacin 750 mg once a day for 5 days or 500 mg once a day for 10 days.

Hospital-Acquired Pneumonia

Figure 1 is an algorithm for treatment of pneumonia in hospitalized patients.

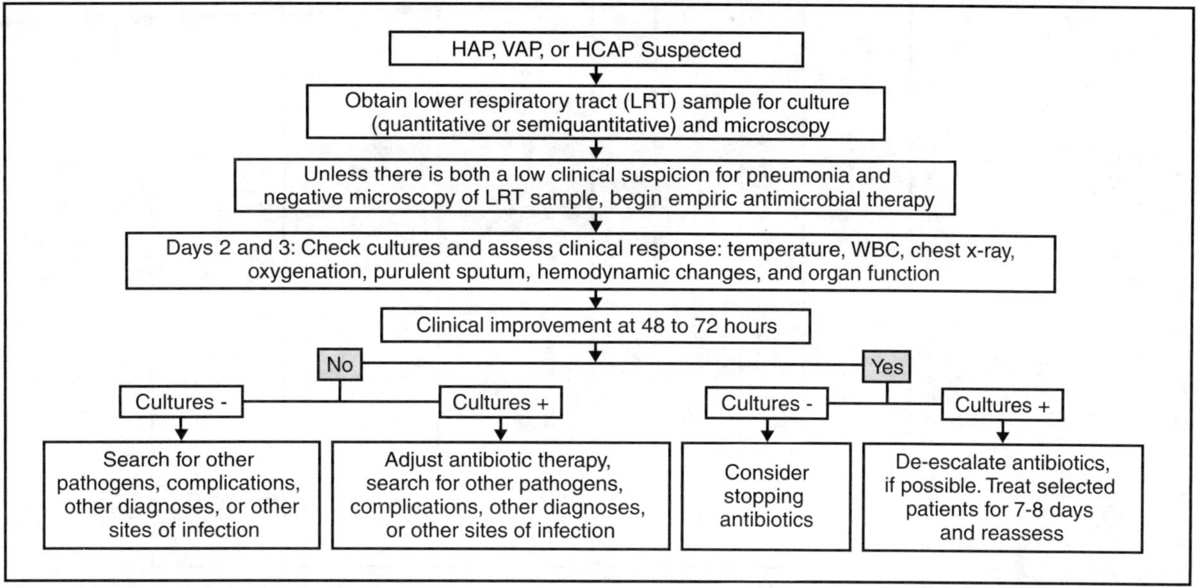

Figure 1: Pneumonia in hospitalized patients. Summary of management strategies for a patient with suspected hospital-acquired pneumonia (HAP), ventilator-associated pneumonia (VAP), or health-care associated pneumonia (HCAP). (*Am J Respir Crit Care Med* 2005;171:388-416.)

Acute Bronchitis

Prodromal URI. Productive mucopurulent cough, rhonchi, sometimes wheezing, no x-ray densities. Often viral or nonbacterial.

Chronic Bronchitis

Coexisting, frequent chronic obstructive pulmonary diseases (chronic bronchitis, emphysema). Cultures not helpful. Irritants may be important. Bronchospasm and inflammation are frequent. Sputum becomes

Location	Primary Diagnosis	Secondary Diagnosis/ Contributing Factors	Pathogens
Lung	pneumonia	neonate	*Chlamydia* group A or B streptococci *H influenzae, S aureus,* *E coli, Pseudomonas*
		infant bronchopneumonia	*Chlamydia*
		empyema pneumatoceles	pneumococci *H influenzae*
		empyema pneumatoceles	*S aureus*
		outpatient ambulatory	*Mycoplasma pneumoniae* *Chlamydia pneumoniae** *S pneumoniae*
	anthrax	mediastinal widening on chest x-ray	*B anthracis*
	severe acute respiratory syndrome (SARS)		viral

*Clarithromycin and dirithromycin not FDA approved for this indication.

more purulent or changes in color or consistency.

Bronchiectasis

Chronic cough, large amounts purulent sputum, some hemoptysis. Rales and rhonchi.

Pneumonia

Pneumococcal: fever, chills, chest pain, cough, rusty sputum, x-ray—lobar infiltration mostly, also bronchial. Culture—sputum, blood. Increased or decreased white blood cell count, left shift.

4

Empiric Choices	Alternatives	Duration	Other Measures/ Comments
erythromycin		10-14 d	
ampicillin + aminoglycoside	carbenicillin/gentamicin; oxacillin/gentamicin	14-21 d	Differentiate from RDS.
erythromycin	azithromycin sulfisoxazole	5 d 14 d	
ampicillin cefuroxime	azithromycin erythromycin chloramphenicol	5 d 10-14 d	Drain empyema.
nafcillin oxacillin	vancomycin*	14-21 d	
clarithromycin azithromycin or doxycycline If *S pneumoniae*, consider alternatives.	If at risk for resistant pathogens: gatifloxacin moxifloxacin levofloxacin telithromycin	5-10 d 1 d**	Cough may continue. Organisms may persist in sputum, even after cure.
ciprofloxacin doxycycline penicillin	levofloxacin ofloxacin or other quinolones	60 days▲	Prophylaxis for subjects exposed to spores. **Not contagious from person to person.**
			Supportive therapy.

* If at risk for MRSA

** Azithromycin extended-release oral suspension formulation, single dose 2 g.

▲Treatment: ciprofloxacin, 400 mg IV q 12 h; doxycycline, 100 mg P.O. q 12 h

▲Prophylaxis: ciprofloxacin, 500 mg P.O. q 12 h; doxycycline, 100 mg P.O. q 12 h

continued on next page

Location	Primary Diagnosis	Secondary Diagnosis/ Contributing Factors	Pathogens
Lung *(continued)*	pneumonia	community adult (bacterial)	*S pneumoniae* *H influenzae* *S aureus** *M pneumoniae* *C pneumoniae* *M catarrhalis* *Legionella* sp *Klebsiella* sp**

* Rule out endocarditis.
** May be seen in patients with substance (eg, alcohol) abuse.

Empiric Choices (parenteral/oral)	Alternatives (parenteral/oral)	Duration	Other Measures/ Comments
if unknown, ceftriaxone + macrolide (azithromycin IV, erythromycin IV) if proven *S aureus* then or oxacillin, nafcillin	If penicillin-allergic, erythromycin, or clindamycin + aminoglycoside or aztreonam; 3rd-generation cephalosporins, piperacillin/ tazobactam* amoxicillin/ clavulanate XR**	7-10 d	In hospitalized patient, obtain sputum. Blood, pleural fluid, or transtracheal aspirate cultures.
If resistant pathogens: vancomycin levofloxacin† gatifloxacin moxifloxacin cefepime	azithromycin*** clarithromycin**** telithromycin▲▲	1-5 d▲ 7-10 d	

* For moderate severity secondary to *H influenzae*.

** Including strains with reduced susceptibility to PCN with MICs of 2 μg/mL.

*** Only for pneumonia of mild severity due to *S pneumoniae* and *H influenzae*, and only for patients who can take oral therapy. The FDA recently approved azithromycin extended release oral suspension formulation, single dose 2 g.

**** Only for *S pneumoniae*.

▲ For oral therapy; 7-10 d for IV followed by oral therapy.

▲▲ For mild to moderate infection.

† Now approved for 750-mg/d x 5 d.

continued on next page

4

Respiratory Tract Infections *(continued)*

Location	Primary Diagnosis	Secondary Diagnosis/ Contributing Factors	Pathogens
Lung *(continued)*	pneumonia	hospitalized patient*	*S pneumoniae* *H influenzae* *Klebsiella* *E coli* *S aureus*** oral flora
			Pseudomonas
		intubated patient	*Pseudomonas* coliforms oral flora

*Guidelines for the management of adults with hospital-acquired, ventilator-associated, or health-care-associated pneumonia. Statement from the American Thoracic Society and Infectious Diseases Society of America. *Am J Resp Crit Care Med* 2005;171:388-416.

**Consider MRSA.

Empiric Choices	Alternatives	Duration	Other Measures/ Comments
3rd-generation cephalosporin + macrolide or quinolones (levofloxacin, gatifloxacin, moxifloxacin) or aztreonam + oxacillin or nafcillin or clindamycin or vancomycin; cefepime piperacillin/tazobactam;	linezolid (for MRSA)	8-14 d	Difficult to define exact etiology. Two antibiotics may be preferable to monotherapy. In hospitalized patient, obtain sputum. Blood pleural fluid, or transtracheal aspirate cultures.
piperacillin or cefepime or ticarcillin/clav. or imipenem + an aminoglycoside or quinolones (ciprofloxacin, levofloxacin*)	piperacillin/ tazobactam + an aminoglycoside or quinolones (ciprofloxacin, levofloxacin*)		Piperacillin or mezlocillin not to be used for *S aureus*
piperacillin/ tazobactam + an aminoglycoside mezlocillin' ticarcillin/clav. aztreonam + imipenem, meropenem, or cefepime aminoglycoside or quinolones (ciprofloxacin, levofloxacin*)		14 d	Some patients are colonized with gram-negative bacilli (GNB); differentiation from infection on clinical grounds necessary.

*Levofloxacin: dose should be 750 mg once a day.

The New Pneumonias

Since the outbreak of legionnaires' disease in Philadelphia, many strains of *Legionella* have been isolated. Increasing fever, pulmonary infiltrates, gastrointestinal disturbances, and renal dysfunction in a normal or compromised host should lead to consideration of *Legionella*, especially with failure to respond to conventional agents.

Occupational exposure may increase awareness. Diagnosis is based on either sputum isolation (rare), im-

Pneumonia in the Immunocompromised Host

Pathogens	Comments	Empiric Choices
Bacteria:		
gram-negative bacilli (GNB) *Serratia* *Acinetobacter* *Pseudomonas*	Necrotizing pneumonia, cavitation.	3rd-generation cephalosporins, or imipenem/cilastatin; piperacillin/tazobactam*; aztreonam, or tobramycin + piperacillin or cefoperazone or ceftazidime ticarcillin/clavulanate quinolones (levofloxacin***, ciprofloxacin) cefepime trovafloxacin**
Fungi:		
Aspergillus	Rapidly progressive necrotizing pneumonia, hemoptysis.	voriconazole amphotericin B lipid preparation of amphotericin B caspofungin
Pseudallescheria boydii	Rapidly progressive necrotizing pneumonia, hemoptysis.	voriconazole miconazole itraconazole
Phycomycetes (*Mucor*)	Rapid cavitation. Pleuritic pain. Hemoptysis. Rhinocerebral infection may occur.	amphotericin B lipid preparation of amphotericin B
Cryptococcus	Diffuse pattern. CNS involvement. Skin lesions may occur.	amphotericin B + 5-flucytosine lipid preparation of amphotericin B fluconazole

* An aminoglycoside should be added when *Pseudomonas* is being treated or is suspected.

** Serious to fatal liver damage has occurred, so safer alternative antimicrobial therapy is recommended, when available.

*** Levofloxacin dose: 750 mg once a day.

munofluorescent staining of sputum, or lung biopsy, as well as rises in serologic titer. Similar syndromes are caused by a variety of agents, ie, Wiga and Pittsburgh pneumonia agent, which have now been characterized as genus *Legionella micdadei.* Other species isolated are: *L bozemanii, L dumoffii, L gormanii, L longbeachae,* and *L wadsworthii.* Therapy with intravenous erythromycin, azithromycin, or tetracycline should be instituted in a patient with pneumonia who fails to respond to conventional agents. Intravenous therapy may be necessary in seriously ill or immunocompromised

Alternatives	Suggested Duration	Other Measures/Comments
	2-4 wk	Difficult to prove the diagnosis since cultures are often contaminated with gram-negative bacilli.
caspofungin* itraconazole* addition of tetracycline may help	unknown	Diagnosis by fiberoptic bronchoscopy or open-lung biopsy. Antigen determination is a promising test. Antibodies not reliable for *Aspergillus.*
	unknown	
	unknown	Transtracheal aspirate or fiberoptic bronchoscopy. CNS involvement common.
itraconazole	unknown	Cryptococcal antigen determination in serum and CSF is important.

*FDA approved for pulmonary and extrapulmonary aspergillosis in patients who are refractory or intolerant to amphotericin B therapy.

continued on next page

patients. Differential diagnosis may include viral, *Mycoplasma*, and *Chlamydia* sp, *Pneumocystis jiroveci* (in the immunosuppressed).

Pulmonary Tuberculosis: May be minimal features. Lassitude, malaise, anorexia, weight loss, fever (especially in afternoon), cough, rales, hemoptysis. Positive tuberculin test—particularly change from negative to positive. Primary tuberculosis, lower lobes,

Pneumonia in the Immunocompromised Host *(continued)*

Pathogen	Comments	Empiric Choices
Fungi *(continued)*		
Histoplasma	Diffuse, nodular, cavitating	amphotericin B and/or itraconazole
Candida	Diffuse or lobar	amphotericin B caspofungin fluconazole lipid preparation of amphotericin B
Nocardia	CNS or bone lesions, usually cavitating pulmonary lesion. Skin often involved.	TMP/SMX linezolid (in vitro)*
Viral:		
herpes simplex herpes zoster		acyclovir**
respiratory syncytial virus (RSV)		ribavirin ± RSV-IgG* (RespiGam)
cytomegaloviruses	Usually diffuse interstitial pattern, miliary.	ganciclovir***
adenoviruses Epstein-Barr virus		

* Not FDA approved for this indication.
** For herpes simplex and herpes zoster (not FDA approved for these indications).
*** For cytomegalovirus (not FDA approved for this indication) but is now approved for prevention of CMV in bone marrow and heart transplantation.

postprimary apical infiltration; cavities. Sputum, gastric, and tracheal washings. ***Klebsiella:*** Associated with debilitation, alcoholism, diabetes, superinfection. Sudden onset, dyspnea, cyanosis, sticky 'currant-jelly' sputum. Lung abscess common. High fatality in untreated cases.

Pseudomonas and ***Proteus:*** Debilitation, superinfection, inhalation therapy. Necrotizing lesions, widespread consolidation. High fatality. **Streptococcal:** Uncommon. Cyanosis, rapid development of pleural effusion. Bloody sputum.

Alternatives	Suggested Duration	Other Measures/Comments
unknown		Complement fixation titer may not rise. Bone marrow, liver, or lung biopsy may be necessary to prove diagnosis.
itraconazole*	unknown	Oral contamination makes sputum culture and fiberoptic brushing unreliable. Antigen assay promising.
tetracycline sulfadiazine erythromycin cycloserine (CNS infection) minocycline	unknown	CAT scan of brain to rule out CNS infection. No serologic test.
ganciclovir** for cytomegaloviruses; experimental use in AIDS and transplant patients.		Often associated with fungal or parasitic infection. CMV—may have viruria or rise in complement fixation titer. Hyperimmune globulin + ganciclovir have been used in bone marrow transplant patients with CMV.

* FDA approved for pulmonary and extrapulmonary aspergillosis in patients who are refractory or intolerant to amphotericin B therapy.

** See package insert for indications, dosages, and toxicities.

continued on next page

Respiratory Tract Infections *(continued)*

Staphylococcal: After viral infection or as superinfection. Initial malaise, headache, cough. Sudden onset, spiking fever, cough, cyanosis, hemoptysis. X-ray often shows air-fluid cavities. Pleural effusion. High leukocytosis. Sputum, pleural fluid culture, and blood culture necessary. Often associated with bacterial endocarditis.

Pneumonia in the Immunocompromised Host *(continued)*

Pathogen	Comments	Empiric Choices
Parasites:		
Pneumocystis jiroveci	Diffuse, may be lobar; respiratory distress. Diagnosis by sputum smear or bronchoscopy.	TMP/SMX or pentamidine
Toxoplasma gondii	CNS symptoms may be present; CAT scan with multiple lesions.	sulfadiazine + pyrimethamine
Strongyloides stercoralis (hyperinfection syndrome)	Associated with gram-negative bacteremia; eosinophilia. Diagnosis: egg and worm in sputum.	thiabendazole ivermectin
Intracellular Bacteria:		
Chlamydia trachomatis	Lobar or diffuse; antibody titer may rise.	doxycycline
Higher Order Bacteria:		
Legionella pneumophila subtypes: *L bozemanii* (Wiga) *L micdadei* (Heba Tatlock Pittsburgh agent) *L dumoffii*, *L gormanii* *L longbeachae* *L wadsworthii*	Often associated with gastrointestinal symptomatology. Renal insufficiency.	erythromycin or doxycycline + rifampin dirithromycin levofloxacin azithromycin* trovafloxacin**

* IV formulation only

** Serious to fatal liver damage has occurred, so safer alternative antimicrobial therapy is recommended, when available.

Mycoplasma: Fever, headache, dry cough. Cough most prominent. Infiltration may be more prominent than physical findings.

Anaerobic oral flora: Fusobacteria, streptococci, *Bacteroides* sp. Underlying and predisposing conditions: alcoholism, seizures, aspiration, chronic onset, fever, foul breath, lower lobes. Consider transtracheal aspiration. Pneumonitis, lung abscess, necrotizing pneumonia, empyema, all possible.

4

Alternatives	Suggested Duration	Other Measures/Comments
atovaquone (for mild to moderate disease) trimetrexate* + leucovorin* clindamycin + pyrimethamine*	3 wk 2-4 wk	May recur in AIDS; prophylaxis may be necessary; serology not perfected.
	not known	Seen in lymphoma, AIDS, and transplant patients (mainly cardiac). Diagnosis serologically or by biopsy. Clindamycin + pyrimethamine being studied in AIDS patients.
	2-7 d	May present with asthma.
erythromycin ofloxacin azithromycin**	2 wk	May occur in normal or immunocompromised adults.
quinolones clarithromycin***	2-4 wk	Not uncommon in renal transplants; look for environmental source; may present as community-acquired pneumonia. For azithromycin, 7-10 d for IV followed by oral therapy.

* See package insert for indications, dosages, and toxicities.
** Dose is 1 g combined with other antibiotics.
*** In vitro only.

Respiratory Tract Infections *(continued)*

Location	Primary Diagnosis	Secondary Diagnosis/ Contributing Factors	Pathogens
Bronchi and lung	bronchiolitis	infantile	Virus—RSV, parainfluenza
Lungs, bronchi, and pleura	tracheobronchitis	adolescent	*M pneumoniae* parainfluenza adenovirus
	acute bacterial exacerbations of chronic bronchitis	chronic, 'smoker's' bronchitis, pollution, viral URI	*H influenzae*—usually nontypable *M catarrhalis* *S pneumoniae*

Empiric Choices	Alternatives	Duration	Other Measures/ Comments
ribavirin (aerosolized monoclonal AB) palivizumab*		 once monthly	Watch for development of secondary bacterial pneumonia.
erythromycin azithromycin clarithromycin none	tetracycline	7-10 d 3-5 d 5-7 d	Cough often persists.
doxycycline TMP/SMX	moxifloxacin gatifloxacin telithromycin levofloxacin cefixime ceftibuten clarithromycin azithromycin cefuroxime axetil cefpodoxime proxetil amoxicillin/ clavulanate loracarbef	3-7 d	Postural drainage, physical therapy. Appropriate bronchodilators. In some patients, consider corticosteroids.

* For prophylaxis of RSV infection in high-risk children.

continued on next page

Respiratory Tract Infections *(continued)*

Location	Primary Diagnosis	Secondary Diagnosis/ Contributing Factors	Pathogens
Lungs, bronchi, and pleura *(continued)*	anaerobic pleuropulmonary disease	aspiration pneumonia (outside hospital)	*Fusobacterium* *Peptostreptococcus* *Bacteroides**
		aspiration pneumonia (in hospital)	*Fusobacterium* *Peptostreptococcus* *Bacteroides** gram-negative bacilli
		lung abscess (admitted from community)	*Fusobacterium* *Peptostreptococcus* *Bacteroides**
		lung abscess (inpatient)	*Fusobacterium* *Peptostreptococcus* *Bacteroides** plus aerobic gram-negative bacilli
	any anaerobic pleuropulmonary disease with empyema		as above

*β-lactamase-producing strains may be resistant to penicillin therapy.

Empiric Choices	Alternatives	Duration	Other Measures/ Comments
clindamycin parenteral penicillin G	piperacillin ampicillin/sulbactam may have role ticarcillin/clavulanate piperacillin/tazobactam amoxicillin/clav.	2-6 wk	Physical therapy
clindamycin + aminoglycoside; ticarcillin/clavulanate piperacillin; 3rd-generation cephalosporins + metronidazole; nafcillin or cefazolin + aztreonam piperacillin/tazobactam cefepime	ampicillin/sulbactam may have role fluoroquinolones gatifloxacin moxifloxacin	2-6 wk	Parenterally, then long oral therapy, 1 to 3 mo.
parenteral penicillin G, or aminoglycoside 3rd-generation cephalosporins* piperacillin/tazobactam	ampicillin/sulbactam piperacillin clindamycin fluoroquinolones gatifloxacin moxifloxacin	4-6 wk	Long time to clear x-ray. Follow-up therapy with P.O. agents for last few weeks.
clindamycin + aztreonam piperacillin/tazobactam	piperacillin/tazobactam + aminoglycoside	2-6 wk	Penicillin V for several months. Cefoxitin only if no *Pseudomonas*. Follow therapy with P.O. agents for last few weeks.
as above piperacillin/tazobactam	as above	4-6 wk	Empyema must be drained surgically.

*May need additional antianaerobic agents.

4

Section 5: Infections of the Cardiovascular System

Acute Infective Pericarditis

Pain (substernal, pleuritic, or precordial) neck, shoulder, back. Pericardial friction rub. ECG—ST elevation early; later, T inversion with no Q waves. Chest x-ray—pleural effusion. Associated pneumonic changes suggest TB. Echocardiogram helpful.

Bacterial Endocarditis

Subacute: Preexistent heart disease, eg, congenital, rheumatic, atherosclerotic, usual. Persistent fever, loss of weight, joint pain, myalgia, anemia. Murmur, petechiae, embolic signs, splenomegaly. Positive blood cultures. Normochromic anemia, urinary casts, pro-

Location	Primary Diagnosis	Secondary Diagnosis/ Contributing Factors	Pathogens
Heart	acute bacterial endocarditis	pneumonia or meningitis	pneumococci (rare)
		narcotic addict, IV catheter	*S aureus* *Pseudomonas* *P cepacia* *Serratia* *Burkholderia*
	subacute bacterial endocarditis	dental procedures colon lesion	*S viridans* *S bovis*
			S faecalis *S milleri* B_6-requiring streptococci

teinuria, microscopic hematuria may be present. Positive rheumatoid factor, if more than 4-6 weeks of symptoms. Echocardiogram to determine if vegetation present.

Acute: History of surgery, instrumentation, narcotic addiction, previous infection elsewhere. High fever, murmurs, emboli, petechiae. Echocardiogram often positive.

Septic Thrombophlebitis

May be associated with cellulitis. Pain, tenderness along course of vein. Associated with indwelling IV catheter. Positive swab for smear and culture. Physical examination may be misleading.

5

Empiric Choices	Suggested Alternatives	Duration	Other Measures/ Comments
penicillin G vancomycin (if penicillin resistant or penicillin allergy)	add ceftriaxone if penicillin resistant	4-6 wk	Supportive, check for congestive heart failure (CHF)
nafcillin or oxacillin + aminoglycoside*; antipseudomonal β-lactam + aminoglycoside, if *Pseudomonas*	cephalosporin + aminoglycoside*, vancomycin for MRSA; daptomycin is under investigation for MSSA and MRSA	4-6 wk	Surgery needed if *Pseudomonas* or *Serratia* species on left side, or CHF, repeated emboli, or uncontrolled infection.
penicillin	ceftriaxone cephalosporin, clindamycin, vancomycin; addition of an aminoglycoside may sterilize valves faster	4 wk	Surgery for CHF or repeated emboli. If *S bovis* isolated, work up GI tract for neoplasia.
penicillin or ampicillin + aminoglycoside	vancomycin + aminoglycoside	4-6 wk	Surgery for CHF or repeated emboli.

*Usually given for up to 5 days.

continued on next page

Infections of the Cardiovascular System *(continued)*

Location	Primary Diagnosis	Secondary Diagnosis/ Contributing Factors	Pathogens
Heart (*continued*)	prosthetic valve endocarditis	early <60 days	*S aureus* MSSA/MRSA *S epidermidis* coliforms *Candida*
		late	*S viridans* *S epidermidis**
	pericarditis		viral
		endocarditis postsurgical trauma	*Staphylococcus* pneumococcus *Streptococcus* *Neisseria* coliforms

*Usually methicillin resistant.

Empiric Choices	Suggested Alternatives	Duration	Other Measures/ Comments
nafcillin or oxacillin + aminoglycoside; if MRSA, then vancomycin, if GNB, 3rd-generation cephalosporin or piperacillin + aminoglycoside		6 wk	Valve usually must be removed. May need to add rifampin for *S epidermidis*, or methicillin-resistant *S aureus* infection.
for *S epidermidis*: vancomycin and/or rifampin and/or gentamicin		6 wk	May need surgery. Rifampin usage for *S epidermidis* or methicillin-resistant *S aureus* infections.
			Supportive only. Steroid usage?
oxacillin or nafcillin + aminoglycoside; if GNB, 3rd-generation cephalosporin or piperacillin + aminoglycoside, if MRSA, then vancomycin	ceftriaxone	4-6 wk	Aspiration. Window drainage. Adjust antibiotic pending culture results.

Section 6: Vascular Infections

Location	Primary Diagnosis	Secondary Diagnosis/ Contributing Factors	Pathogens
Vein	septic thrombo-phlebitis	secondary to catheterization	*S aureus* *Pseudomonas* coliforms
		hyperalimentation	*Candida*, other bacteria
		postpartum abortion	anaerobes *Bacteroides* clostridia *Streptococcus*

Empiric Choices	Alternatives	Suggested Duration	Other Measures/ Comments
antistaphylococcal penicillin or vancomycin + aminoglycoside; cefepime if GNB, 3rd-generation cephalosporin or piperacillin + aminoglycoside or aztreonam	cephalosporin ciprofloxacin if *Pseudomonas* For MRSA, consider if vancomycin intolerant or failure: linezolid, or quinupristin/dalfopristin or daptomycin	as needed 10-21 d	Remove catheter. Perform Gram stain. Ligation may be needed. Avoid prolonged indwelling catheters. Rule out endocarditis.
if septic, amphotericin B or caspofungin; if bacterial, antibiotics		unknown	Vein may need to be removed. With candidiasis, check fundus to rule out ophthalmitis. Late sequelae; metastatic foci may occur, ie, arthritis.
clindamycin + aminoglycoside or aztreonam; piperacillin or mezlocillin or 3rd-generation cephalosporin; if septic, add aminoglycoside or aztreonam; piperacillin/tazobactam	chloramphenicol cefoxitin cefotetan	as needed	Anticoagulation. Remove septic focus. May need inferior vena cava plication/ligation.

6

Environmental factors, stool smears essential for differential diagnosis.

Intestinal and Anorectal Infection in Homosexual Men

Enteric and anorectal infections occurring in homosexuals may be caused by the following organisms: *Shigella, Salmonella, Campylobacter fetus* subspecies *jejuni, Entamoeba histolytica, Giardia lamblia, Neisseria gonorrhoeae, Neisseria meningitidis, Chlamydia trachomatis, Treponema pallidum.* (See specific infection for recommendations for therapy.)

Toxigenic diarrhea

E coli—Traveler's. Little fever. No polys in stool. Fluid replacement.

Shigellosis

Lower abdominal pain, diarrhea. Fever, myalgias. Stool smear shows polys. Sigmoidoscopy: positive.

Location	Primary Diagnosis	Secondary Diagnosis/ Contributing Factors	Pathogens
Mouth	Vincent's infection (angina)	necrotizing gingivitis	fusobacteria *Bacteroides* spirochetes
	candidiasis	thrush	*Candida albicans*
Stomach	gastritis gastric ulcer		*H pylori*

Giardiasis

Bloating, foul, fatty stools. Nonspecific complaints, weight loss.

Salmonellosis

May have enteritislike picture; stools nonbloody, few polys in smear. Low-grade fever. Blood cultures should be performed.

Cholera

Geographic history. Sudden, severe diarrhea, rice-water stool. Dehydration, acidosis, hypokalemia, hypotension. Positive stool cultures.

Others

Vibrio parahaemolyticus—shellfish. ***V vulnificus***—may present with septicemia and skin lesions. ***Campylobacter fetus***—subsp, *jejuni*. ***Yersinia*** species associated with arthritis.

Typhoid Fever

Gradual onset, malaise, headache prominent, cough, often constipation. Fever with slow pulse. Rose spots rare, splenomegaly, slight abdominal distention. Leukopenia, positive stool, blood culture.

7

Empiric Choices	Alternatives	Duration	Other Measures/ Comments
ampicillin/sulbactam amoxicillin/clav. penicillin G	clindamycin, tetracycline piperacillin/tazobactam	1-3 wk	Analgesics. Improve oral hygiene. Dental referral.
nystatin mouthwash	clotrimazole troches, P.O. ketoconazole, P.O.		Gargle and swallow.
clarithromycin with: • omeprazole or • ranitidine + bismuth citrate	bismuth + tetracycline + metronidazole: if this triple therapy is used, see Duration	2 wk with antisecretory drug	An additional 2 weeks of antisecretory therapy is recommended.

continued on next page

Gastrointestinal Infections *(continued)*

Acute Cholecystitis

Associated with gallstones, nausea, vomiting, right upper quadrant tenderness and pain. Fever, leukocytosis. Sonography helpful.

Peritonitis

Prior abdominal disease. Pain, vomiting, fever. Rigidity, rebound tenderness. Distention, paralytic ileus, toxicosis. Leukocytosis. X-ray—gas and fluid collections. Abdominal tap sometimes useful.

Diverticulitis

Secondary to diverticulosis (asymptomatic). Lower quadrant pain, fever, constipation. Left lower quadrant mass. Leukocytosis. X-ray diverticula, narrowing especially in sigmoid.

Location	Primary Diagnosis	Secondary Diagnosis/ Contributing Factors	Pathogens
Intestines	acute bacterial gastroenteritis	shigellosis	*Shigella*
		salmonellosis	*Salmonella enteritidis*
			Vibrio parahaemolyticus
		other agents	*Campylobacter* invasive *E coli*
			rotavirus
	yersiniosis	food contamination	*Yersinia enterocolitica* *Y pseudotuberculosis*
	traveler's diarrhea	turista—prevent with doxycycline or bismuth subsalicylate (Pepto-Bismol)	*E coli*, toxin producing
	cholera		*Vibrio cholerae* El Tor vibrio

GI Ulcer Disease/
***H pylori* infection**

The NIH has issued treatment recommendations for *H pylori* infections associated with duodenal or gastric ulcers. Therapy was recommended for those patients with either initial symptoms or for those with recurrent disease. In vitro studies revealed that certain agents were active against *H pylori.* Clarithromycin was the most active agent when compared with other macrolides, β-lactams, and metronidazole.

A prospective, double-blind, randomized, placebo-controlled trial was carried out giving omeprazole 40 mg once daily for 28 days plus either clarithromycin 500 mg three times daily or placebo for 1 to 14 days. Results at 4-6 weeks revealed that the clarithromycin-omeprazole (C-O) regimen had a bacteriologic eradication rate of 83% vs 1% for the omeprazole-placebo combination.

Empiric Choices	Alternatives	Duration	Other Measures/ Comments
ciprofloxacin ofloxacin, ampicillin, TMP/SMX, tetracycline		1 wk	Many resistant to ampicillin and some tetracyclines.
ciprofloxacin ofloxacin, ampicillin,* amoxicillin*	TMP/SMX	1 wk	Treat only seriously ill patients—the elderly, infants, or immunocompromised. Association with marijuana.
fluid replacement		1 wk	Shellfish
erythromycin ciprofloxacin ofloxacin, ampicillin	TMP/SMX	1 wk	Fluid replacement
fluids		1 wk	
gentamicin	ciprofloxacin doxycycline chloramphenicol IV	as needed	May mimic inflammatory bowel diseases. Often associated with arthritis.
fluid replacement, ciprofloxacin rifaximin (200 mg q.d.)	tetracycline ampicillin ofloxacin TMP/SMX	5 d 3 d	Do not use intestinal sedatives, eg, diphenoxylate, opiates.
doxycycline	ciprofloxacin TMP/SMX	3 d	Fluid replacement IV—rapid. Also P.O. if IV is not possible.

*Antibiotics may prolong carrier state and select resistant strains.

continued on next page

7

Gastrointestinal Infections
(continued)

Ulcer healing rates were essentially equal for the two regimens, 100% vs 99%. However, follow-up duodenal ulcer recurrence rates at 6 months were statistically different: 4% for the C-O regimen vs 55% for the omeprazole-placebo regimen ($P<.001$). Ulcer recurrence rates at 12 months were also markedly different, 6% for C-O vs 76% for omeprazole-placebo. Differences were noted in toxicity between the two groups, being greater in the C-O group; 'taste perversion'

Location	Primary Diagnosis	Secondary Diagnosis/ Contributing Factors	Pathogens
Intestines *continued*	typhoid fever		*Salmonella typhi* *S paratyphi*
	GI inflammation caused by anthrax	diarrhea	*B anthracis*
	giardiasis		*Giardia lamblia*
	duodenal ulcer		*H pylori*
	diverticulitis		Enterobacteriaceae anaerobes

and tongue discoloration were the most common adverse effects in the C-O group. Other therapies have included drug combinations such as omeprazole, clarithromycin, and metronidazole, or bismuth, tetracycline, and clarithromycin.

Triple therapy with bismuth, metronidazole, and tetracycline has been suggested.* If metronidazole was taken previously, then clarithromycin was suggested as an alternative; an antisecretory drug was also recommended.

Empiric Choices (if seriously ill)	**Alternatives**	**Duration**	**Other Measures/ Comments**
ampicillin, chloramphenicol IV, ciprofloxacin ofloxacin	TMP/SMX ceftriaxone	14-21 d	Resistance to chloramphenicol common in Central and South America.
ciprofloxacin** doxycycline**	possibly other quinolones	60 days	Sepsis may occur
furazolidone metronidazole		1 wk	Parasite seen in stool or in duodenal aspirate.
clarithromycin with: • omeprazole or amoxicillin or • ranitidine + bismuth citrate	bismuth + tetracycline + metronidazole: if this triple therapy is used, see Duration	2 wk with anti-secretory drug	An additional 2 weeks of anti-secretory therapy is recommended.
ampicillin P.O.*** tetracycline P.O.*** amoxicillin/ clavulanate P.O.***	if patient is severely ill, aminoglycosides or aztreonam + ampicillin or clindamycin or ampicillin/sulbactam or cefoxitin or cefotetan; 3rd-generation cephalosporins + metronidazole piperacillin/tazobactam quinolones (used in conjunction with metronidazole) cefepime plus metronidazole tigecycline	as needed	Fluid replacement. Rest the intestine. Do not use cefoxitin or imipenem with aztreonam.

* Drug therapy. *N Engl J Med* 1995;333:984-991.

** Treatment: ciprofloxacin, 400 mg IV q 12 h; doxycycline, 100 mg IV q 12. Prophylaxis: ciprofloxacin, 500 mg P.O. q 12 h; doxycycline, 100 mg P.O. q 12 h.

*** In patients less seriously ill treated at home.

continued on next page

Gastrointestinal Infections *(continued)*

Location	Primary Diagnosis	Secondary Diagnosis/ Contributing Factors	Pathogens
Rectum, anus	anorectal abscess	perirectal abscess	Enterobacteriaceae *Bacteroides* enterococci
Appendix	acute appendicitis: perforation	perforation	organisms as above
Gall Bladder	cholecystitis	acute, no obstruction	*E coli* *Klebsiella* enterococci
		chronic, obstruction	coliforms anaerobes *Clostridium* (in diabetics)
	cholangitis		*E coli* *Klebsiella* enterococci

Empiric Choices (if seriously ill)	Alternatives	Duration	Other Measures/ Comments
clindamycin + aminoglycoside or aztreonam or ciprofloxacin or ofloxacin* or ampicillin/sul. or piperacillin or mezlocillin or 3rd-generation cephalosporin, cefoxitin** or cefotetan** metronidazole + aminoglycoside or aztreonam piperacillin/tazobactam tigecycline	meropenem	as needed	Surgical intervention is primary therapy.
ampicillin/sulbactam or mezlocillin, or 3rd-generation cephalosporin, cefoxitin** or cefotetan** clindamycin or metronidazole + aminoglycoside or aztreonam piperacillin/tazobactam cefepime plus metronidazole tigecycline	imipenem/ cilastatin meropenem ertapenem	as needed	Surgery and antibiotics for perforation.
cephalosporin (cefuroxime) cefepime plus metronidazole piperacillin/tazobactam tigecycline		as needed	Fluids, surgery later.
cephalosporin (cefuroxime) or piperacillin/tazobactam tigecycline			
cephalosporin or piperacillin, or ampicillin/sulbactam piperacillin/tazobactam tigecycline	clindamycin + aminoglycoside or aztreonam quinolones	as needed	Fluids; adjust therapy pending blood cultures.

* Ciprofloxacin and ofloxacin are not active against anaerobes.
** Do not use aztreonam with cefoxitin or with cefotetan.

continued on next page

Gastrointestinal Infections *(continued)*

Location	Primary Diagnosis	Secondary Diagnosis/ Contributing Factors	Pathogens
Peritoneum	peritonitis	secondary to small bowel leak	*E coli* *Klebsiella* enterococci anaerobic flora
		from colonic lesion	*E coli* *B fragilis* *Klebsiella* *Enterobacter*
		intra-abdominal abscess, fistula	
Liver	abscess	secondary to gastro-intestinal infection, often cryptic	coliforms anaerobes *B fragilis* enterococci

Empiric Choices (if seriously ill)	Alternatives	Duration	Other Measures/ Comments
3rd-generation cephalosporin or cefoxitin or cefotetan or ampicillin/sulbactam cefepime or ciprofloxacin + metronidazole tigecycline	imipenem/ cilastatin meropenem	as needed	Gram stain. Adjust therapy pending blood cultures.
cefepime or ciprofloxacin + metronidazole clindamycin + aminoglycoside or aztreonam or piperacillin/tazobactam metronidazole + aminoglycoside or aztreonam or ampicillin/sulbactam tigecycline	meropenem cefoxitin or cefotetan or chloram-phenicol IV + amino-glycoside* ertapenem imipenem	as needed	Surgical drainage. Adjust therapy pending blood cultures.
ciprofloxacin + metronidazole tigecycline			
3rd-generation cephalosporins, aminoglycosides + clindamycin or metronidazole + aminoglycoside cefoxitin** or cefotetan** quinolones or piperacillin/tazobactam	imipenem meropenem	as needed	Aspiration or surgery is usually necessary.

*Chloramphenicol and aminoglycoside may be antagonistic.
**Do not use aztreonam with cefoxitin or with cefotetan.

7

Section 8: Urinary Tract Infections

Lower Urinary Tract Infection

Urgency, frequency, dysuria, suprapubic pain, occasionally fever. White cells in urine, bacteria on unspun specimen. Symptoms may not distinguish between upper and lower tract disease.

Urethral Syndrome (Women)

Dysuria, pyuria, bacterial count is less than 10^5. Etiology: usually *Chlamydia*.

Upper Urinary Tract Infection

Chills, fever, frequency, urgency, dysuria, pain/tenderness in costovertebral angle. Malaise, nausea, anorexia, pyuria, red cells, granular and white cell casts, mild proteinuria, bacteria on unspun urine specimen, antibody-coated bacteria may be present.

Location	Primary Diagnosis	Secondary Diagnosis/ Contributing Factors	Pathogens
Kidney and tract	lower urinary tract infection	asymptomatic bacteriuria associated with recurrent exacerbations	*E coli* *Klebsiella* *Proteus* *Enterobacter*
		cystitis, no underlying pathology	*E coli*

Chronic Urinary Tract Infection

May be asymptomatic. Urine unrevealing—has few white cells, but bacteria present. Leukocytes.

Urinary Tract Tuberculosis

Dysuria, frequency, nocturia, malaise, fatigue, night sweats. 'Sterile' pyuria, hematuria. IVP may make diagnosis. Culture concentrated AM urine.

Prostatitis

Acute: Perineal or low back pain, dysuria, frequency, urgency, fever, pyuria, bacteriuria, rarely purulent urethral discharge. Tender, swollen prostate.

Chronic: Prostate feels normal, perhaps harder, may be either normal or enlarged.

Empiric Choices (if seriously ill)	Alternatives	Duration	Other Measures/ Comments
amoxicillin ampicillin or TMP/SMX, or cephalosporin ciprofloxacin* Treat young or pregnant patients as for cystitis. Cannot use sulfonamides in last trimester.	ofloxacin*	7-14 d 3-7 d	Recheck bacterial count at 2 weeks and 12 weeks. Investigate possible anatomic defects. If *Proteus*, look for stones.
TMP/SMX ampicillin** ciprofloxacin**	oral cephalosporin** ofloxacin* loracarbef*** cefpodoxime proxetil gatifloxacin* levofloxacin**	1 d 7 d▲ 3 d	Many cured with 3 g dose of amoxicillin. TMP/SMX, tetracyclines, and quinolones contraindicated in pregnancy.

* Quinolones not to be used in children or in pregnant women.

** Drugs are not approved for use in pregnancy.

*** For uncomplicated pyelonephritis caused by *E coli.*

▲ In uncomplicated infection in women without obstruction, diabetes, or pregnancy, may use single dose or 1-day therapy.

continued on next page

Urinary Tract Infections *(continued)*

Location	Primary Diagnosis	Secondary Diagnosis/ Contributing Factors	Pathogens
Kidney	upper urinary tract infection	pyelonephritis: community-acquired	*E coli* *P mirabilis*
		hospital-acquired	*Klebsiella* *Enterobacter* *Pseudomonas* enterococci
	perinephric abscess		*S aureus* *E coli*
Prostate	prostatitis	acute	*E coli* *Klebsiella* *Enterobacter* *Proteus* *S aureus* *N gonorrhoeae* *C trachomatis*
		chronic	*E coli* *Klebsiella* *Enterobacter* *Proteus* enterococci *Pseudomonas*
Epididymis	epididymitis orchitis	young, usually sexually transmitted	*Chlamydia*
		older patients	*E coli* *Proteus*

Empiric Choices (if seriously ill)	Alternatives	Duration	Other Measures/ Comments
ampicillin or cephalosporin ciprofloxacin* gatifloxacin* (*E coli* only) cephalosporins or piperacillin, mezlocillin, ticarcillin/ clavulanate, TMP/SMX piperacillin/ tazobactam** cefepime	TMP/SMX cephalosporin or ofloxacin* aminoglycosides or aztreonam, 3rd-generation cephalosporin or ciprofloxacin*	14 d 7 d 10 d 14 d	Repeat culture at 2 days. If fever persists, check for abscess or obstructed kidney. Community-acquired *E coli* is usually sensitive; hospital-acquired is often resistant. May need 6 weeks of therapy.
cephalosporins piperacillin/ tazobactam ticarcillin/ clavulanate	imipenem meropenem aminoglycoside quinolones?*	14-28 d	Percutaneous or surgical drainage. Follow-up therapy based on culture results.
quinolones 3rd-generation cephalosporins piperacillin/ tazobactam or ampicillin + aminoglycosides	TMP/SMX	14 d ofloxacin therapy should be given for 6 wk***	Encourage fluids. Analgesics, bed rest, sitz baths. Rarely, culture positive.
quinolones doxycycline TMP/SMX erythromycin	ciprofloxacin if *Pseudomonas*†	14-28 d ofloxacin therapy should be given for 6 wk***	Treat complicating infections. Long-term therapy may be indicated. Associated with recurrent chronic urinary infections or inadequate acute therapy.
ceftriaxone doxycycline levofloxacin ofloxacin	erythromycin ciprofloxacin	10-14 d 7-28 d 10 10 d	Bed rest, scrotal elevation; treat sexual partners. Treat according to urine culture.

* Quinolones not to be used in children or in pregnant women.

** See piperacillin package insert for appropriate dosage.

*** Therapy may be initiated with ofloxacin IV, with a switch to P.O. when patient's condition dictates.

† Not approved.

8

Section 9: Gynecologic Infections

Infective Vaginitis

Pruritus, dyspareunia, leukorrhea. Discharge excessive, malodorous.

Pelvic Inflammatory Disease

Gonorrhea, *Chlamydia*. Lower cramping, abdominal pain and adnexal tenderness, fever, etc. Abscess development possible. Recurrent pelvic pain, pelvic masses, dysmenorrhea, dyspareunia. Fatigue, anemia, infertility.

Location	Primary Diagnosis	Secondary Diagnosis/ Contributing Factors	Pathogens
Salpinges Adnexae Uterus	sexually transmitted diseases		*N gonorrhoeae* and/or *C trachomatis*

Venereal Infections:

Gonorrhea (Male)

Purulent urethral discharge, dysuria, positive smear. Epididymitis, prostatitis, proctitis (male homosexual). Fever, arthritis, dermatologic lesions. Secondary complications. Positive smear and culture.

Nongonococcal Urethritis

Slight urethral secretion, exacerbations and remissions. Dysuria not frequent, periurethral pruritus common. Discharge may be serous, mucopurulent, or purulent. No bacteria on smear. Postgonococcal complaints continue. *Chlamydia* usual agent.

Empiric Choices*	Alternatives*	Other Measures/ Comments
Uncomplicated: 1) ceftriaxone, 125 mg IM 2) cefixime, 400 mg P.O. x 1 3) ciprofloxacin, 250 mg P.O. x 1 4) ofloxacin, 400 mg P.O. x 1 5) cefpodoxime proxetil, 200 mg P.O. x 1 6) cefuroxime axetil, 1 g P.O. x 1 7) azithromycin, 2 g P.O. 8) gatifloxacin, 400 mg P.O. x 1	For disseminated gonococcal infection: 1) ceftriaxone, 1 g/d IM or IV until improvement, then continue for 24-48 h ceftizoxime or cefotaxime, 1 g IV q 8 h until improvement, then continue for 24-48 h	Avoid intercourse. Gonococcal resistance to tetracycline and TMP/SMX is increasing in developing countries. The sexual partner should be treated.
All of the above are plus tetracycline, 500 mg, P.O., q.i.d. for 7 days or doxycycline, 100 mg, b.i.d. for 7 days	2) if β-lactam allergy, spectinomycin, 2 g IM b.i.d. q 24-48 h, then add: cefixime 400 mg P.O. b.i.d. x 7 d, or ciprofloxacin 500 mg P.O. b.i.d. x 7 d**	
Alternate therapy for gonorrhea: spectinomycin, 2 g IM q 12 h until improvement, followed by tetracycline or doxycycline	All patients should be treated for chlamydial infections, ie, doxycycline, 100 mg b.i.d. x 7 d, or ofloxacin, 300 mg b.i.d. x 7 d (In pregnancy, use erythromycin base 500 mg q.i.d. x 7 d)	

* For further treatment options, see STD treatment guidelines in *MMWR* 1993;42:RR-14.

** Ciprofloxacin resistance has been reported.

continued on next page

Gynecologic Infections *(continued)*

Syphilis

Primary chancre stage: nonpainful sore; second-degree stage: mucocutaneous, sore throat, many diverse lesions, lymphadenopathy; third-degree stage: neurosyphilis, cardiovascular, gumma, etc. Diagnosis—primary darkfield microscopy. Screening—VDRL, ART. More specific—FTA-ABS.

Location	Primary Diagnosis	Secondary Diagnosis/ Contributing Factors	Pathogens
Salpinges **Adnexae** **Uterus** (*continued*)	pelvic inflammatory disease (PID) salpingitis or endometritis	intrauterine device	coliforms *Bacteroides* *Chlamydia* *N gonorrhoeae* *C trachomatis* *Mycoplasma hominis*

Lymphogranuloma Venereum

Unnoticed ulcerative lesion. Inguinal lymphadenopathy, draining sinuses. Proctitis, strictures (females, homosexual males). Systemic involvement occasionally. Positive Frei's test, complement fixation, raised serum globulin.

Chancroid

Macule breaks down to ulcer, unilateral adenitis, multiple lesions. Mixed infection common. Positive culture, chancroid skin test. Balanitis, phimosis. Buboes can become fluctuant.

Empiric Choices*	Alternatives*	Other Measures/ Comments
For PID: If hospitalized, then parenteral treatment with: a) cefoxitin, 2 g IV q 6 h or cefotetan, 2 g IV b.i.d., + doxycycline, 100 mg P.O. or IV b.i.d. Both agents are given for at least 48 h after patient clinically improves. Then doxycycline, 100 mg P.O. b.i.d. for 10-14 d. b) clindamycin, 900 mg IV q 8 h + gentamicin, loading dose IV or IM (2 mg/kg body weight), followed by 1.5 mg/kg q 8 h. Both agents are given for at least 48 h after patient improves; doxycycline, 100 mg P.O. b.i.d. for 10-14 d, or clindamycin, 450 mg q.i.d. for 10-14 d. c) ampicillin/sulbactam, 3 g IV q 6 h + doxycycline 100 mg P.O. or IV q 12 h, or ofloxacin, 400 mg IV q 12 h, or levofloxacin, 500 mg q.d. IV with or without metronidazole, 500 mg IV q 8 h d) piperacillin/tazobactam, 3.375 g q 6 h. If ambulatory, then: either, cefoxitin 2 g IM + probenecid 1 g P.O., or ceftriaxone, 250 mg IM or equivalent cephalosporin + doxycycline, 100 mg P.O. b.i.d. for 10-14 d, or tetracycline, 500 mg q.i.d. for 10-14 d.		If abscesses are present or if patient fails to respond, surgery may be necessary.

*For further treatment options, see STD treatment guidelines in *MMWR* 2002;51:RR-6.

continued on next page

9

Scabies

Itching, pustules, superficial burrows.

Herpes Simplex Type 2

Vesicular lesion. Painful, recurrent. Much more common than syphilis; must be differentiated.

Location	Primary Diagnosis	Secondary Diagnosis/ Contributing Factors	Pathogens
Salpinges **Adnexae** **Uterus** *(continued)*	endometritis		*Bacteroides* *Clostridium perfringens* *E coli* enterococci group A or B streptococci
	Chlamydia infection		*C trachomatis*

Empiric Choices*	Alternatives*	Other Measures/ Comments
penicillin** or piperacillin/ tazobactam or 3rd-generation cephalosporins, clindamycin or cefoxitin*** + aminoglycoside or aztreonam or ampicillin/sulbactam ticarcillin/clavulanate		D and C; may need hysterectomy. Hyperbaric O_2 may be helpful in clostridial infections. Disseminated intravascular coagulation (DIC) often occurs. Endometritis from other causes may require surgery, and if associated with pelvic vein thrombosis, anticoagulation therapy.
tetracycline† 500 mg q 6 h for 7 d or doxycycline† 100 mg b.i.d. for 7 d ofloxacin† 300 mg b.i.d. x 7 d azithromycin 1 g stat	erythromycin base: 500 mg q.i.d. for 7 d; sulfisoxazole: 500 mg q.i.d. for 10 d	Treat interim sex partners.

* For further treatment options, see STD treatment guidelines in *MMWR* 2002; 51:RR-6.

** Use penicillin for clostridial infections; since these infections are often mixed, additional agents are necessary.

*** Do not use aztreonam with cefoxitin.

† Should not be given to pregnant women.

continued on next page

9

Location	Primary Diagnosis	Secondary Diagnosis/ Contributing Factors	Pathogens
Vagina	vaginitis		*Candida albicans*
			Trichomonas vaginalis
	bacterial vaginosis		*Gardnerella vaginalis* *M hominis* *Mobiluncus* sp *Prevotella* sp
	nongonococcal urethritis (NGU)		*Chlamydia trachomatis* *Ureaplasma urealyticum*

Empiric Choices	Alternatives	Duration	Other Measures/ Comments
fluconazole, 150 mg P.O. x 1 dose clotrimazole, 1 % cream 5 g intravaginally x 7-14 d miconazole, 200 mg vaginal suppository, 1 x 3 d terconazole cream, 5 g intravaginally HS x 3 d	gentian violet, topical		Check for diabetes.
metronidazole, 500 mg b.i.d. x 7 d	metronidazole, 2 g as 1 dose		Treat male consort; metronidazole, 2 g, as 1 dose, if required.
metronidazole, 500 mg, P.O., b.i.d. for 7 d	clindamycin, 2% cream 5 g intravaginally at bedtime x 7 d, or metronidazole, 0.75% gel 5 g intravaginally b.i.d. x 5 d, or clindamycin, 300 mg P.O. b.i.d. x 7 d***		Necessity for routine treatment of male sex partners is unknown. Organism often associated with other anaerobes.
doxycycline,* 100 mg b.i.d. x 7 d azithromycin** 1 g stat	erythromycin, 500 mg, P.O., q.i.d. for 7 d, or erythromycin succinate, 800 mg P.O. q 6 h x 7 d, or erythromycin base, 250 mg q.i.d. x 14 d, or erythromycin ethylsuccinate, 400 mg q.i.d. x 14 d levofloxacin, 500 mg q.d. x 7 d		Treat sexual partner. In pregnancy, use only erythromycin.

* Should not be given to pregnant women.
** Approved for *C trachomatis* but not for *U urealyticum*.
***For pregnant women, may use metronidazole 250 mg P.O. t.i.d. x 7 d.

continued on next page

9

Location	Primary Diagnosis	Secondary Diagnosis/ Contributing Factors	Pathogens
Genitourinary Tract	chlamydia infections		*Chlamydia trachomatis*
	syphilis*	early syphilis: less than 1 year's duration	*Treponema pallidum*
		syphilis of more than 1 year's duration (except neurosyphilis; includes cardiovascular syphilis)	*Treponema pallidum*
		neurosyphilis	*Treponema pallidum*

*For further treatment options, see STD treatment guidelines in *MMWR* 2002; 51:RR-6.

Empiric Choices	Alternatives	Duration	Other Measures/ Comments
azithromycin, 1 g P.O. x 1 dose or doxycycline,* 100 mg b.i.d. x 7 d	ofloxacin,* 300 mg P.O. b.i.d. x 7 d or erythromycin base, 500 mg P.O. q.i.d. x 7 d, or erythromycin ethylsuccinate, 800 mg P.O. q.i.d. x 7 d azithromycin 1 g stat		
benzathine penicillin G, 2.4 million U, IM x 1	if penicillin-allergic, ceftriaxone: 1 g IM/IV q.d. x 8-10 d tetracycline,* 500 mg q 6 h or doxycycline,* 100 mg b.i.d., or erythromycin base, 500 mg q 6 h	14 d 14 d 14 d	Check male consort.
same dose, once a week for 3 wk	doxycycline*: 100 mg P.O. b.i.d. x 28 d tetracycline* 500 mg q 6 h erythromycin 500 mg q 6 h	28 d 28 d	No published studies documenting efficacy for drugs other than penicillin.
18-24 million U/d aqueous penicillin, IV, in divided doses for 10-14 d followed by 2.4 million U benzathine penicillin IM weekly for 3 doses	aqueous procaine penicillin 2.4 million U/d IM + probenecid, 500 mg q.i.d. for 10 d followed by benzathine penicillin regimen, 2.4 million U. IM weekly for 3 doses		None of these regimens has been adequately studied. Penicillin-allergic, then tetracycline,* 500 mg P.O. q.i.d. for 28 d.

*Tetracycline, doxycycline, ofloxacin should not be given to pregnant women.

continued on next page

Gynecologic Infections *(continued)*

Location	Primary Diagnosis	Secondary Diagnosis/ Contributing Factors	Pathogens
Perineum Penis	lympho-granuloma venereum		*Chlamydia*
	chancroid		*Haemophilus ducreyi*
	granuloma inguinale		*Calymmatobacterium granulomatis*
	herpes simplex 2 initial episode		herpes simplex 2 herpes simplex 1 (5%-10%)

Empiric Choices	Alternatives	Duration	Other Measures/ Comments
doxycycline,* 100 mg b.i.d. x 21 d	erythromycin, 500 mg P.O. q.i.d. x 21 d, or sulfisoxazole, 500 mg P.O. q.i.d. x 21 d	14 d	Rectal stricture problem in females, LGV-CF test available. Relapse common.
azithromycin, 1 g** P.O. x 1 or ceftriaxone 250 mg IM 1 dose or erythromycin, P.O. 500 mg q.i.d. for 7 d ciprofloxacin, 500 mg P.O. b.i.d. x 3 d			Buboes, pustular lesions, organisms may look gram-positive.
doxycycline 100 mg P.O. b.i.d. x 3 wk TMP/SMX-DS: b.i.d. x 3 wk	erythromycin: 500 mg P.O. q.i.d. x 3 wk ciprofloxacin: 750 mg P.O. q.d. x 3 wk azithromycin: 1 g P.O. each wk x 3 wk	10-14 d	May coexist with other venereal infections.
acyclovir, P.O., 400 mg, t.i.d. x 7 d, acyclovir IV used for AIDS or other immunocompromised patients famciclovir 250 mg t.i.d. x 7-10 d valacyclovir 1,000 mg b.i.d. x 7 d For AIDS patients: valacyclovir,*** 500 mg b.i.d. x 5 d		7-10 d	Avoid intercourse during blister phase.

* Doxycycline should not be given to pregnant women.

** Males only.

*** Thrombotic thrombocytopenic purpura/hemolytic uremic syndrome (TTP/HUS), in some cases resulting in death, has occurred in patients with advanced HIV disease and also in allogeneic bone marrow transplant and renal transplant recipients in clinical trials of valacyclovir at doses of 8 g/d. This was not observed in clinical trials in immunocompetent patients.

continued on next page

9

Gynecologic Infections *(continued)*

Location	Primary Diagnosis	Secondary Diagnosis/ Contributing Factors	Pathogens
Perineum Penis *(continued)*	herpes simplex, recurring infections		
	herpes simplex, suppressive therapy		

Empiric Choices	Alternatives	Duration	Other Measures/ Comments
acyclovir, 400 mg P.O. t.i.d. x 5 d, or acyclovir, 200 mg P.O. 5 times a day for 5 d, or acyclovir, 800 mg P.O. b.i.d. x 5 d, or famciclovir, 125 mg P.O. b.i.d. x 5 d, or valacyclovir, 500 mg P.O. b.i.d. x 3-5 d, or valacyclovir, 1 g q.d. x 5 d			
acyclovir 400 mg b.i.d. P.O.*, or famciclovir, 250 mg b.i.d. P.O.**, or valacyclovir, 1 g q.d. P.O.**			

*Safety has been documented for up to 6 years.

**Safety has been documented for up to 1 year.

9

Section 10: Central Nervous System Infections

Brain Abscess

May follow infection at a contiguous site (eg, mastoiditis, frontal sinusitis). Focal or progressive neurologic signs. Raised intracranial pressure—headache, papilledema, localizing neurologic signs. Mild fever. CAT scan, EEG, brain scan, angiography. Lumbar puncture of little help.

Cranial Epidural Abscess

Follows chronic sinus infection, neurologic defects slight, x-ray, EEG, CAT scan, surgery required.

Spinal Epidural Abscess

Backache, sudden pain, fever, sudden sensory motor loss; myelography, surgery required. *S aureus* most common organism.

Subdural Empyema

Complication of osteomyelitis after sinusitis, high fever, stiff neck, elevated CSF pressure, many WBCs. Use CAT scan to diagnose. *S aureus*, anaerobes are most common infecting organisms. Surgery essential.

Meningitis

Headache, fever, mental abnormalities, nuchal rigidity, positive Kernig's and Brudzinski's sign. Lumbar puncture—white cells, decreased glucose, increased protein, gram stain.

Location	Primary Diagnosis	Secondary Diagnosis/ Contributing Factors	Pathogens
Brain	abscess	endocarditis and following CNS surgery	*S aureus*
			Pseudomonas
		Anaerobic infection elsewhere. Otic infection. Congenital cyanotic heart disease	*Bacteroides* *Actinomyces* anaerobic streptococci *Proteus*
	shunt infection		*S epidermidis*

Types: a) **Purulent**—pyogenic organisms; b) **Granulomatous**—tuberculosis, fungi, syphilis; c) **Viral**; d) **Neonatal**—postsepticemia, lacking typical sign.

Meningococcal Meningitis

Fever, headache, confusion, delirium, convulsions. Petechial or hemorrhagic rash. Shock and intravascular clotting. Neurologic signs: do LP, blood culture. Usually no local infection preceding onset. Prophylaxis for close contacts, ie, intimate family members, day-care centers. Prophylaxis should be started immediately.

Pneumococcal Meningitis

Preceding infection in sinuses, ears, lungs. Symptoms similar to meningococcal meningitis.

Haemophilus influenzae Meningitis

Mostly in children under 8 years old. Similar features to other purulent meningitis. Diagnosis by CSF culture, countercurrent immunoelectrophoresis.

Tuberculous Meningitis

Gradual onset, fatigue, anorexia. Headache, vomiting, convulsions, coma. Nuchal rigidity. TB focus elsewhere (not always). PPD may be negative. LP: neutrophils initially, later lymphocytes predominate. Sugar de-

Empiric Choices	Alternatives	Duration	Other Measures/ Comments
nafcillin or vancomycin oxacillin + 3rd- or 4th-generation cephalosporin		3-6 wk	Aspiration or surgical drainage. Adjust agents pending culture results.
ceftazidime piperacillin + tobramycin cefepime	gentamicin, amikacin	3-6 wk	Aspiration or surgical drainage. Adjust agents pending culture results.
high-dose penicillin G, metronidazole (not approved)	cefotaxime or ceftriaxone + metronidazole	4-6 wk	Aspiration or surgery usually required.
adults: vancomycin + rifampin children: ceftriaxone or cefotaxime + vancomycin		until cleared	Shunt removal may be necessary for cure.

10

continued on next page

creased. Markedly elevated protein suggests CSF block.

Cryptococcal Meningitis

Immunosuppressed patient. Headache, personality changes, low-grade fever. LP: sugar depressed, lymphocytes. Obtain cryptococcal antigen.

Location	Primary Diagnosis	Secondary Diagnosis/ Contributing Factors	Pathogens
Meninges	meningitis in neonate		group B streptococci *E coli* *Listeria* *Pseudomonas*
	meningitis in child under 10 years of age		*H influenzae* meningococcus pneumococcus
	adult meningitis		meningococcus pneumococcus *H influenzae*
			S aureus *Pseudomonas* Enterobacteriaceae

Rocky Mountain Spotted Fever
Occurs in children or adults. Tick exposure in 80%, often when camping; usually between spring and fall. Headache, rash—may mimic meningitis. LP: lymphocytes, normal glucose. Obtain complement fixation titers for diagnosis.

Empiric Choices	Alternatives	Duration	Other Measures/ Comments
ampicillin* or penicillin G + aminoglycoside, cefotaxime, or ceftriaxone	penicillin G	21 d	
ceftriaxone or cefuroxime + vancomycin + dexamethasone	meropenem For severe PCN allergy: vancomycin + TMP/SMX	10-14 d	If *H influenzae* is resistant to ampicillin and patient is penicillin allergic, then give chloramphenicol IV. For penicillin-resistant strains of *S pneumoniae*, combination therapy with vancomycin, ceftriaxone or cefotaxime, plus rifampin.
24 million U penicillin G or 12 g ampicillin* ceftriaxone 4 g** cefotaxime 12 g**	chloramphenicol, cefuroxime, erythromycin if penicillin-allergic	10-14 d	Arteritis associated with pneumococci. Meningococcemia with disseminated intravascular coagulation may occur. For penicillin-resistant strains, combination therapy with vancomycin, ceftriaxone or cefotaxime, plus rifampin.
nafcillin or oxacillin for *S aureus*; cefotaxime or ceftizoxime; ceftriaxone for some gram-negative bacteria; for *Pseudomonas*, ceftazidime or piperacillin	aztreonam may be given for *Pseudomonas* as additional IV therapy ciprofloxacin***	2-3 wk	May need intrathecal gentamicin for *Pseudomonas*. Adjust therapy by culture.

* Ampicillin not effective against β-lactamase-producing strains.
** Maximum dose.
*** Has been used in refractory cases for gram-negative infections. Penetration into CNS not reliable.

continued on next page

Central Nervous System Infections *(continued)*

Location	Primary Diagnosis	Secondary Diagnosis/ Contributing Factors	Pathogens
Meninges *(continued)*	meningitis adult/child	normal	free-living amoeba *Naegleria*
		immunocompromised	*Listeria*
			Cryptococcus
			Toxoplasma gondii

Empiric Choices	Alternatives	Duration	Other Measures/ Comments
amphotericin B, rifampin + pentamidine, 5-FC, TMP/SMX		14-28 d, or until clinically better	Associated with swimming in fresh water. Purulent meningitis—negative gram stain; organisms seen unstained on wet preparation of CSF. Poor prognosis.
ampicillin + aminoglycoside	TMP/SMX, chloramphenicol IV tetracycline		Relapse may occur. Chloramphenicol IV has been associated with failures.
amphotericin + 5-FC or fluconazole		4-8 wk until patient is afebrile and cultures are negative	Amphotericin, 0.6 mg/kg/d, + 5-FC, 150 mg/kg/d; fluconazole, 200 mg/d; disease may occur in normal patients.
sulfadiazine, 1-1.5 g P.O. q 6 h + pyrimethamine, 75-100 mg P.O. + folinic acid 10-15 mg/d P.O. x 3-6 wk	TMP/SMX 5/25 mg based on TMP dose IV/P.O. q 12 h x 30 d		Diagnosis on wet preparation of CSF, or rising titer.

10

continued on next page

Central Nervous System Infections *(continued)*

Location	Primary Diagnosis	Secondary Diagnosis/ Contributing Factors	Pathogens
Meninges *(continued)*	tuberculous meningitis		*M tuberculosis*
	prophylaxis: close contact (family) with meningococcal meningitis		*N meningitidis*
	prophylaxis: close contact (family)		*H influenzae*
	Rocky Mountain spotted fever child/adult	tick exposure, camping; rash, headache	*R rickettsii*

Empiric Choices	Alternatives	Duration	Other Measures/ Comments
isoniazid + rifampin pyrazinamide ethambutol*	cycloserine	9 mo to 1 yr (optimal duration of therapy not determined)	Steroids needed if intracranial pressure increases. Must check antibiotic sensitivities and adjust regimen; use drugs that penetrate CNS. Monitor liver function.
adults: rifampin 600 mg P.O. q.d. x 2 d children: rifampin 10-20 mg/kg P.O. q.d. x 4 d or ciprofloxacin** 500 mg	minocycline: P.O. 100 mg b.i.d. x 5 d for patients >8 yr ceftriaxone: 250 mg IM for adults, 125 mg IM for children <15 yr		If sulfa-sensitive, use sulfonamide.
rifampin may be helpful; dosage as above		4 d	
doxycycline; if severely ill, use IV chloramphenicol		10-14 d	May occur without rash; disseminated intravascular coagulation (DIC) may occur.

* Therapy may be adjusted after induction period of 2 months; monitor for liver toxicity.
** Not to be used in children or pregnant women.

10

Section 11: Infections of the Eye

Blepharitis
Inflamed lid margins. Nonulcerative (seborrheic)—ulcerative (staphylococcal). Scaling, ulceration, loss of lashes. Irritation, burning.

Stye (Hordeolum)
Staphylococcus abscess. Tender lid. Internal or external. Pain, swelling, cellulitis.

Conjunctivitis
Bacterial: purulent discharge.
Viral: watery discharge, scant exudate, often from swimming pools.
Trachomal: common in Asia, Africa. Bilateral inflammation, itching, watery discharge, scant exudate. Increased exudate with exacerbations. Keratitis and blindness.

Dacryocystitis
Infection of lacrimal sac. Unilateral, secondary to nasolacrimal duct obstruction. Pain, tenderness, erythema. Purulent discharge.

Location	Primary Diagnosis	Secondary Diagnosis/ Contributing Factors	Pathogens
Eyelid	blepharitis	ulcerative	*S aureus*
	stye	hordeolum	*S aureus*
Eye	conjunctivitis		*S aureus* *S pneumoniae* *E coli* *Proteus*
	chlamydal conjunctivitis of newborn		*Chlamydia trachomatis*

Endophthalmitis
Pain, loss of vision, chemosis, eyelid swelling, rapid purulent involvement. Constitutional symptoms usually severe.
Fungal: symptoms less severe. May lose eye.
Keratitis (corneal ulcer): emergency.
Pneumococcal: gray ulcer, well-defined. Redness, lacrimation, pain, photophobia.
***Pseudomonas* or *Proteus*:** virulent, posttrauma, rapid spread, perforation, blue-green pigmentation.

Herpes simplex virus: severe infection, producing dendritic ulcers and geographic ulcers (recurrent infections); ruptured vesicles stain green with fluorescein dye. Herpetic keratitis, if allowed to go untreated or treated unsuccessfully, could lead to partial loss of sight and/or blindness.

Ophthalmia Neonatorum
Bacterial: 2-5 days postpartum.
Chlamydial: 5-10 days postpartum.

Empiric Choices*	Alternatives	Duration	Other Measures/ Comments
ophthalmic erythromycin or chloramphenicol ointment to eyelids	sulfacetamide, neomycin, polymyxin B	as needed	Control scalp seborrhea, rarely need to use oxacillin or nafcillin or cephalosporin injectable.
nafcillin or oxacillin (systemic)	cephalosporin, clindamycin piperacillin/ tazobactam	as needed	Use antibiotics only for advanced cases (cellulitis, etc). Topicals of no use. Incision and hot compress useful.
ophthalmic topical polymyxin B, bacitracin, neomycin topical moxifloxacin ophthalmic 0.5% base	topical gentamicin or tobramycin	7 d	
topical 0.5% erythromycin ophthalmic ointment, or 1% tetracycline drops/ointment, q 4 h for 2 wk	erythromycin syrup, 50 mg/kg/d, in divided doses, q 6 h for 2 weeks (preferred therapy)		

*All topical eye ointments are *ophthalmic* ointments only.

continued on next page

11

Infections of the Eye *(continued)*

Location	Primary Diagnosis	Secondary Diagnosis/ Contributing Factors	Pathogens
Eye *(continued)*	gonococcal ophthalmia		*Neisseria*
		trachoma	*Chlamydia*
	dacryocystitis	inflamed lacrimal gland	*S aureus* *Streptococcus* *S pneumoniae* *Pseudomonas*
	endophthalmitis		*S aureus* *Pseudomonas* *Klebsiella* *S pneumoniae* *Streptococcus* *Meningococcus*
			fungal *Candida* *Aspergillus*
	chorioretinitis		cytomegalovirus

Empiric Choices*	Alternatives	Duration	Other Measures/ Comments
ceftriaxone IM/IV		1 dose	Saline irrigation of eyes.
doxycycline P.O.**	erythromycin	1-3 wk	
according to smear culture, nafcillin or oxacillin, cephalosporin	aminoglycoside	as needed	Relief of nasolacrimal duct obstruction needed for cure.
vancomycin + amikacin; subconjunctival and/or intravitreal injection***	cephalosporin + gentamicin or other amino-glycosides	as needed	Blood cultures + Gram stain critical. Vitrectomy may be necessary.
amphotericin, IV; intravitreal amphotericin B has been given**	5-flucytosine (for *Candida* sp)	as needed	Vitrectomy may be necessary.
ganciclovir or foscarnet or valganciclovir	cidofovir + probenecid		Usually occurs in immuno-compromised host. Diagnosis by stain and culture of urine and/or a rising complement fixation titer.

* All topical eye ointments are *ophthalmic* ointments only.

** Doxycycline should not be given to pregnant women or children.

*** Ophthalmic injections of antibiotics should be carried out only by ophthalmologists.

continued on next page

Infections of the Eye *(continued)*

Location	Primary Diagnosis	Secondary Diagnosis/ Contributing Factors	Pathogens
Eye *(continued)*	keratitis	corneal ulcer	*N gonorrhoeae*
			S pneumoniae
			S aureus
			Pseudomonas
			herpes simplex
			fungal
		inclusion conjunctivitis	*Chlamydia*

Empiric Choices*	Alternatives	Duration	Other Measures/ Comments
systemic penicillin + topical tetracycline or chloramphenicol eyedrops; if penicillin-resistant, cefotaxime, cefuroxime or ceftriaxone	sulfacetamide	7 d	Smear urgent, culture needed.
cefazolin + tobramycin or gentamicin	erythromycin (topical)	7 d	
subconjunctival** antistaphylococcal antibiotics	erythromycin (topical)	until improved	
tobramycin or gentamicin + piperacillin or ticarcillin (topical)	ciprofloxacin or ofloxacin (topical)	until improved	Parenteral therapy also necessary.
trifluridine (topical)	ara-A IDU (topical)	7-14 d	These results vary.
amphotericin B	natamycin (topical)	until improved	May require surgery and subconjunctival and topical use of a polyene antibiotic.
ciprofloxacin or ofloxacin (topical)	erythromycin (topical) sulfacetamide (topical)	as needed	Oral sulfonamide or tetracycline may be necessary.

* All topical eye ointments are *ophthalmic* ointments only.
** Ophthalmic injections of antibiotics should be carried out only by ophthalmologists.

11

Section 12: Musculoskeletal Infections

Thomas M. File Jr, MD

Myositis

Myositis, or pyomyositis, is an acute bacterial infection of skeletal muscle. Although common in tropical countries, it had been uncommon in temperate regions, but its incidence is increasing in association with the HIV pandemic, other chronic illnesses, and IV drug use. Other risk factors for developing pyomyositis include trauma, poor general health (malnutrition, recent viral or parasitic infections), and chronic illness. The presumed pathogenesis involves prior bacteremia, which may be asymptomatic. An association between *Toxocara canis* infection (visceral larva migrans) and staphylococcal pyomyositis has been proposed.

The most common pathogen in pyomyositis is *Staphylococcus aureus*, followed by *Streptococcus* species, Enterobacteriaceae, *Pseudomonas*, anaerobes (including *Clostridium* sp), and *Mycobacterium tuberculosis*. Clinical and epidemiologic characteristics are similar regardless of the causative pathogen. However, group A streptococci are being reported more frequently, especially in patients with diabetes in North America, and may have a more aggressive clinical course. *Clostridium* species may be associated with gas gangrene.

Diagnosis is based on clinical findings of fever with local pain and swelling. Conventional x-rays of affected areas may show subcutaneous gas, and sonography may reveal an increase in muscle mass and hypoechoic collections, but more specific and accurate imaging studies such as CT and MRI are now used. It is essential to obtain samples from a muscular abscess for Gram staining and culture. Therapy involves appropriate antimicrobials as well as surgical incision and drainage.

Osteomyelitis

Osteomyelitis can be categorized by the origin of the infection. It usually arises by hematogenous spread, by contiguous spread from soft tissue infection, or by local inoculations after trauma or surgery. The etiology varies with each type, but *S aureus* is the most common pathogen. Osteomyelitis arising from hematogenous spread tends to occur in children and older adults because of the particulars of growing bones in children and an increase in risk factors for bacteremia in adults (eg, central lines, injection drug use, UTIs). The long bones of the femur, tibia, and humerus are most often involved in children, while the vertebrae, sternoclavicular bone, and sacroiliac bones are common in adults.

The signs and symptoms vary with the acuteness of illness, but typically include bone pain, tenderness, warmth, and swelling. Routine laboratory tests are nonspecific. The erythrocyte sedimentation rate (ESR) is usually elevated. Radiologic tests are important in the evaluation of patients with suspected osteomyelitis. Plain films generally require 2 to 3 weeks before bone changes are evident. CT and MRI are more sensitive and specific for showing bone infection. Three-phase bone scan is often used in evaluating osteomyelitis. It has an estimated sensitivity of almost 95% and a high specificity if the plain films are normal and there is no known bone abnormality. However, any process that results in increased bone turnover will show up as 'positive' in a bone scan that is indistinguishable from osteomyelitis. These findings can occur with posttraumatic injury, after surgery, in diabetic feet, septic arthritis, noninfectious inflammatory bone disease, healed osteomyelitis, and Paget's disease. The gold standard for diagnosis is bone biopsy with histopathologic examination and positive culture. Therapy is appropriate antimicrobial therapy (usually for 6 weeks) and may require surgical debridement of necrotic bone, particularly for chronic osteomyelitis.

Septic Arthritis

Most cases of bacterial arthritis arise from hematogenous spread but less commonly can occur from trauma or during joint injection or arthroscopy. Virtually any microbe can cause joint infection, but *S aureus* and streptococci are most common.

Septic arthritis usually presents with an acutely swollen and painful joint. The knee is most commonly involved. Other causes of monoarticular pain and swelling include trauma, crystal-induced arthritis, and reactive arthritis. Gonococcal arthritis commonly presents with migratory polyarthritis and tenosynovitis.

The definitive test of bacterial arthritis is identification of the pathogen in synovial fluid. Synovial fluid cell count, Gram stain, and culture are therefore paramount to establishing the diagnosis. Therapy requires appropriate antimicrobials and adequate joint drainage.

Infection of prosthetic joints occurs in 0.5% to 2.0% of replacements. These infections can be categorized according to the time of onset after implantation: early onset (within the first 3 months) are usually caused by *S aureus* or gram-negative bacilli; delayed onset (3 to 24 months) is usually caused by less virulent organisms such as coagulase-negative *Staphylococcus*; and late onset (>24 months) is typically associated with hematogenous seeding (eg, gram-negative bacilli associated with a UTI). Treatment of prosthetic joint infections usually involves surgical debridement (two-stage replacement arthroplasty is associated with best success rate) followed by a long course of IV antibiotics based on the susceptibility of the offending pathogen.

12

Musculoskeletal Infections *(continued)*

Osteomyelitis

Acute Septic: Fever, malaise, pain, tenderness, swelling. Limitation of motion of adjacent joint. X-ray positive—only after 2-4 weeks. Elevated erythrocyte sedimentation rate (ESR). Culture blood, aspirate from bone. Bone scan.

Septic Arthritis

Fever, pain in joint, swelling, difficulty with motion, aspiration; polymorphonuclears present, decreased sugar; gram stain (may be negative), culture aerobically and anaerobically. No need for intra-articular antibiotics.

Chronic: Follows fractures. Pain, edema, tenderness, sinus tracts present. X-ray usually positive.

Lyme Arthritis

Typical rash of erythema chronicum migrans. Often associated with systemic syndrome, ie, CNS complications, myocarditis. Causal agent is a spirochete; disease is transmitted by tick (*Ixodes dammini*) bite. Treatment with tetracycline is recommended; penicillin for CNS involvement and arthritis.

Location	Primary Diagnosis	Secondary Diagnosis/ Contributing Factors	Pathogens
Muscle	pyomyositis	trauma, HIV, injection drug use	*S aureus*
	clostridial myositis	gas gangrene	*C perfringens* other clostridial strains
	anaerobic myositis	gas may be present	anaerobic streptococci *Bacteroides*

Other Causes
Syphilis, brucellosis, typhoid, fungal (coccidioidomycosis, histoplasmosis, etc).

Viral Arthritides
Have been noted with mumps, rubella, hepatitis, and, recently, parvovirus infections.

Tuberculosis
Onset insidious. Spine most common area. Later bone destruction, limitation of movement, axial skeletal deformity, sinus formation, x-ray not specific. Aspiration of culture and biopsy.

Anaerobic Cellulitis
Gas in tissue, foul odor, little swelling/exudate.

Necrotizing Fasciitis
Fever, acute onset, muscle necrosis. May be aerobic or anaerobic.

Gas Gangrene
Pain, edema in the region of the wound. Brown exudate, skin discoloration. Blebs often present. Crepitations on palpation. X-ray may show gas. Smear for diagnosis. Systemic toxicity major—shock, hemolysis.

Empiric Choices	Alternatives	Duration	Other Measures/ Comments
nafcillin or oxacillin (vancomycin if MRSA)	cephalosporins vancomycin	until improved	Surgical debridement or aspiration.
high-dose penicillin G + clindamycin	ceftriaxone clindamycin doxycycline	until improved	Debridement most important. Polyvalent antitoxin of doubtful benefit. Hyperbaric oxygen helpful.
penicillin G + clindamycin piperacillin/tazobactam ampicillin/sulbactam	metronidazole carbapenem	until improved	Debridement.

12

continued on next page

Musculoskeletal Infections *(continued)*

Location	Primary Diagnosis	Secondary Diagnosis/ Contributing Factors	Pathogens
Bone	osteomyelitis (acute)	neonate	*S aureus* group A streptococci
			Haemophilus
		child/adult	*S aureus*
		postsurgical or contiguous spread from lower extremity ulcer	*S aureus* *Streptococcus* *Pseudomonas* coliforms anaerobes
	osteomyelitis (chronic)	postsurgical, foreign body, trauma	*Staphylococcus* *Pseudomonas* other gram-negative bacilli (GNB)

Empiric Choices	Alternatives	Duration	Other Measures/ Comments
nafcillin or oxacillin or cephalosporin	clindamycin vancomycin	6 wk	Antibiotic based on culture.
ampicillin* or ampicillin/sulbactam	2nd- or 3rd-generation cephalosporin chloramphenicol		
nafcillin or oxacillin (vancomycin if MRSA)	cephalosporin clindamycin, vancomycin	6 wk	May require surgery.
piperacillin/ tazobactam imipenem meropenem	ciprofloxacin or levofloxacin + clindamycin	6 wk	Drainage, appropriate agent continued. Base definitive antimicrobial therapy on susceptibility tests.
must obtain bone culture and treat accordingly ciprofloxacin if P.O. therapy is considered		3-6 wk parenterally, then up to 6-12 mo, P.O. in some cases	Drainage culture often inaccurate; need bone aspirate. Surgery usually necessary for cure.

*Not effective against β-lactamase-producing strains.

continued on next page

Musculoskeletal Infections *(continued)*

Location	Primary Diagnosis	Secondary Diagnosis/ Contributing Factors	Pathogens
Joint	infective (septic) arthritis	neonate	*S aureus* *Streptococcus* coliforms
		children	*S aureus* *H influenzae* *Streptococcus*
		adult Assuming no risk of seeding from other infection site (eg, UTI)	*S aureus* streptococci
		venereal history or contact	gonococcus, including penicillinase-producing *N gonorrhoeae* (PPNG)
		nosocomial	*S aureus* (if nosocomial, MRSA likely) *E coli* *Proteus* *Pseudomonas*
	special organisms	tuberculosis	*M tuberculosis*
		brucellosis	*B abortus*
		salmonella	*S choleraesuis* and other species in immunocompromised
		Lyme arthritis	*Borrelia burgdorferi*

Empiric Choices	Alternatives	Duration	Other Measures/ Comments
nafcillin or oxacillin (use vancomycin if MRSA is a concern) 3rd-generation cephalosporin	vancomycin + 3rd-generation cephalosporin or gentamicin	until improved	Drain hip if involved.
nafcillin or oxacillin or vancomycin (use vancomycin if MRSA is a concern) + 3rd-generation cephalosporin	3rd-generation cephalosporin (+ vancomycin if MRSA)	2-4 wk	Drain hip if involved.
nafcillin or vancomycin (if risk for MRSA)	cephalosporin clindamycin	2-4 wk	
cefotaxime, ceftriaxone, cefuroxime	ciprofloxacin	10-14 d	Tap joint, remove fluid.
vancomycin + cefepime or piperacillin	vancomycin + ciprofloxacin, levofloxacin, or aztreonam	as needed	Selection based on culture data. Drain hip.
isoniazid + rifampin + pyrazinamide	base on susceptibility	9-12 mo	Immobilization not required. Culture sensitivity needed.
doxycycline or tetracycline + gentamicin or streptomycin	TMP/SMX	6 wk	
ampicillin* ceftriaxone	TMP/SMX gentamicin ciprofloxacin	6 wk	
doxycycline 100 mg P.O. q 12 h amoxicillin 500 mg P.O. q 8 h	penicillin or ceftriaxone IV for CNS and arthritis	28 d	Systemic involvement, ie, CNS and myocarditis may occur. Serologic studies prove diagnosis.

*Resistance has been reported.

12

Section 13: Skin and Soft-Tissue Infections

Thomas M. File Jr, MD

Infections of the skin and related structures are among the most common disorders treated by physicians and range from mild pyodermas to life-threatening, necrotizing infections. In the United States, skin infections represent the fourth most common infection that results in outpatient visits in the United States (the top three are all respiratory tract infections—upper respiratory tract infection, otitis media and externa, and lower respiratory tract infections and influenza). Cellulitis is a common cause for admission to hospitals, with a rate of 129 per 100,000 population.

Skin and skin structures provide an initial major barrier for pathogens between humans and their environment, but many potential insults, such as injuries, may disrupt this barrier. In addition, several local or systemic diseases can interrupt skin integrity, such as local trauma, pressure ulcers, and disorders with impaired arterial or venous blood flow. The break in the integrity of the epidermis and deeper layers of the soft tissue allows microorganisms that may be colonizing the skin to become pathogenic.

A myriad of microbes may cause skin and soft tissue infections, but the most common are *Staphylococcus aureus* and *Streptococcus pyogenes.* The manifestations of skin infections are readily detected because inflammatory changes are easily recognizable by the patient.

Infections of the skin and soft tissue can be classified as primary pyodermas; infections associated with underlying conditions of the skin; and necrotizing infections. Primary cutaneous infections of the skin (eg, folliculitis, furunculosis, impetigo, cellulitis, erysipelas) usually occur in the absence of underlying conditions. They are usually caused by a single organism, most commonly *S aureus* or *S pyogenes*, and can usually be treated with local management or oral antimicrobials. Secondary infections develop in association with preexisting lesions (eg, surgical or traumatic wounds, ulcers), which serve as portals of entry for pathogens. Secondary infections are frequently polymicrobial. Necrotizing soft tissue infections (eg, necrotizing fasciitis) are also often found in association with underlying conditions. They are often life threatening and require expeditious recognition and intervention (usually surgical and IV antimicrobials) for optimal patient outcome.

Community-onset (also referred to as community-acquired or community-associated) methicillin-resistant *Staphylococcus aureus* (CO-MRSA) has emerged as a significant and common cause of community skin infections in the past several years. Until recently, MRSA was usually limited to hospitalized patients. However, outbreaks of skin infections caused by CO-MRSA have occurred among prison inmates, injection drug users, gay men, participants in contact sports, and children. There are now enough cases of patients without these risk factors that CO-MRSA needs to be considered in all patients with skin infections. This has increased the importance of obtaining cultures of even mild skin infections. CO-MRSA strains tend to be less resistant to non-β-lactam antimicrobials than hospital-acquired MRSA strains and almost always contain a novel type IV *Staphylococcus* cassette chromosome (SCC) *mec* gene. In addition, many of these strains have been found to contain the gene for Panton-Valentine leukocidin (PVL), a toxin that has been associated with clinical features of serious disease.

In general, CO-MRSA strains are usually susceptible in vitro to trimethoprim/sulfamethoxazole, minocycline, or doxycycline, and often to the fluoroquinolones, although pockets of fluoroquinolone resistant strains exist. In addition, they are often susceptible to clindamycin but the emergence of resistance during therapy has been reported, especially in erythromycin-resistant strains; thus, an erythromycin-induction test (D-test) should be performed on such isolates to determine the presence of in vitro inducible resistance.

Toxic Shock Syndrome

Toxic shock syndrome (TSS) is a multisystem illness that may be caused by exotoxin-producing *S aureus* or *S pyogenes*. Strains of *S aureus* elaborate TSS toxin-1 (TSST-1) or related exotoxins, and certain strains of *S pyogenes* produce pyrogenic exotoxins that are associated with TSS. These toxins can act as 'superantigens' and may activate a much larger proportion of T-cells than do conventional peptide antigens, resulting in excessive production of various cytokines. These cytokines, in turn, are believed to be responsible for most of the manifestations of TSS.

The source of infection is often the skin (particularly for *S pyogenes*) but may include vaginal colonization (associated with tampon use), the respiratory tract, or osteomyelitis for *S aureus.* Symptoms include high fever, hypotension, diffuse erythematous rash, and multiple organ involvement that may rapidly progress to severe and irreversible shock. Mortality is <5% from staphylococcal TSS; for TSS associated with *S pyogenes*, it is 20% to 40%. In addition, about 50% of cases caused by *S pyogenes* are bacteremic, and 50% have necrotizing fasciitis. In contrast, TSS associated with *S aureus* is more likely to be associated with desquamation of skin in the later stages of disease. Diagnosis is made clinically and by isolating the organism. Treatment includes antimicrobials, intensive support, and expeditious surgical debridement. Intravenous immunoglobulin (IVIG) may be of benefit.

Skin and Soft-Tissue Infections *(continued)*

Erysipelas
Superficial cellulitis. Edema, raised border circumscribed.

Human Bites
Associated with oral anaerobes, *Eikenella*. Rapidly progressive infections.

Animal Bites
Check for rabies.

Cellulitis
Less circumscribed, deeper lymphatic involvement.

Impetigo
Macular vesicles, crusts, caused by group A streptococci. Bullous impetigo, both *S aureus* and group A streptococci involved.

Location	Primary Diagnosis	Secondary Diagnosis/ Contributing Factors	Pathogens
Skin	cellulitis	trauma (often minor) to skin	group A or group B, C, G streptococci *S aureus*
		lower extremity cellulitis associated with chronic ulcer	group A streptococci *S aureus* gram-negative bacilli anaerobes
		fresh water injury	*Aeromonas hydrophila*
		salt water injury	*Vibrio vulnificus*

Toxic Shock Syndrome

Toxic shock syndrome (TSS) is an acute febrile illness usually occurring during menstruation. Has been associated with high-absorbency tampons. Symptoms include hypotension, shock, erythrodermic desquamation, myalgias, sore throat, vomiting, diarrhea, and toxic encephalopathy. The etiology is a toxin produced by *S aureus*. Infection with *S pyogenes* has produced a similar clinical picture, with addition of frequent bacteremia and necrotizing fasciitis.

Treatment: fluid replacement, vasopressors, removal of tampon, drainage of any abscess, and administration of a β-lactamase-resistant penicillin or cephalosporin.

Empiric Choices	Alternatives	Duration	Other Measures/ Comments
If not severe, oral therapy: dicloxacillin, cephalexin, cefadroxil, amoxicillin/clavulanate. If CO-MRSA is a concern (see text): TMP/SMX (but does not cover β-streptococci), minocycline, doxycycline, clindamycin (if not inducible resistance). If IV therapy: nafcillin, oxacillin, cefazolin. If MRSA is a concern: vancomycin, linezolid, daptomycin	Oral therapy: macrolide, clindamycin, levofloxacin, moxifloxacin IV therapy: vancomycin, linezolid, daptomycin	clinically determined usually 10 d (one study found 5 d effective for uncomplicated infection)	Surgical debridement may be required.
ampicillin/sulbactam, piperacillin/tazobactam, ertapenem, imipenem meropenem Add vancomycin if concern for MRSA (can also consider linezolid or daptomycin)	tigecycline*, clindamycin + ciprofloxacin or levofloxacin; add vancomycin if concern for MRSA (can also consider linezolid or daptomycin)	clinically determined	Debridement.
fluoroquinolones	imipenem, aminoglycoside		
fluoroquinolones, ceftazidime cefepime	doxycycline		

*Effective for polymicrobial infections, including MRSA, but not for *Pseudomonas* and less effective for *Proteus* sp.

continued on next page

Skin and Soft-Tissue Infections *(continued)*

Folliculitis

Hairy areas, pustules.

Acne Vulgaris

Pustules, papules, cysts, comedones. Face, neck, back. Can persist to adulthood.

Location	Primary Diagnosis	Secondary Diagnosis/ Contributing Factors	Pathogens
Skin *(continued)*	necrotizing fasciitis		group A streptococci *S aureus*
			polymicrobial (anaerobes and aerobes)
	impetigo		group A streptococci *S aureus*
	bites	human animal	anaerobes *P multocida* (cat or dog) *Capnocytophaga canimorsus* (dog) viridans *Streptococcus* *S aureus* *Eikenella* (human)
	furunculosis		*S aureus* (MSSA or MRSA)
	recurrent furunculosis	check for nasal or perianal carrier	*S aureus*

Furunculosis

Boils, carbuncles. Painful follicular abscesses. Avoid excessive manipulation.

Fungal Infections

Superficial skin lesions—tinea. Diagnosis by direct microscopy, UV light, stained smear, culture.

Empiric Choices	Alternatives	Duration	Other Measures/ Comments
penicillin or nafcillin + clindamycin; for MRSA use vancomycin	cephalosporin clindamycin	clinically determined	Surgery mandatory.
piperacillin/tazobactam imipenem, meropenem, ertapenem	ciprofloxacin or levofloxacin + clindamycin or metronidazole		
Topical: mupirocin Oral: penicillin for group A streptococci; if *S aureus,* dicloxacillin (TMP/SMX, minocycline, doxycycline if CO-MRSA)	macrolide clindamycin cephalosporin	clinically determined	In neonatal patients, can be serious.
ampicillin/sulbactam if IV selected or amoxicillin/clav. for P.O. therapy	clindamycin + levofloxacin or ciprofloxacin; cefoxitin, cefotetan, tigecycline	clinically determined	Clean carefully. Check status of tetanus immunization.
dicloxacillin, nafcillin, or oxacillin, but often not needed (local drainage often adequate)	cephalosporin If concern for CO-MRSA: TMP/SMX, minocycline, doxycycline	clinically determined	Incision and drainage. Antibacterial soap, eg, hexachlorophene. Avoid excessive manipulation.
If nasal culture positive, nasal mupirocin Oral therapy: dicloxacillin or TMP/SMX + rifampin	cephalexin + rifampin	10 d	

continued on next page

Skin and Soft-Tissue Infections *(continued)*

Location	Primary Diagnosis	Secondary Diagnosis/ Contributing Factors	Pathogens
Skin *(continued)*	acne vulgaris		*P acnes*
	erysipelas		group A streptococci
	toxic shock	hypotension, high fever, often associated with highly absorbent tampon usage	*S aureus* toxin
		associated with varicella, NSAID use, necrotizing fasciitis	*S pyogenes*
	septic wound	postoperative	*S aureus* (most common) group A streptococci coliforms *Serratia* *Pseudomonas* enterococci anaerobes (if surgery involving GI tract)
		traumatic	*S aureus* group A streptococci coliforms *C perfringens* *C tetani* *Pseudomonas* if puncture wound (especially through tennis shoe)

Empiric Choices	Alternatives	Duration	Other Measures/ Comments
tetracycline, minocycline, topical clindamycin	erythromycin retinoic acid for severe cystic acne	clinically determined	Diet may play no role in treatment. Avoid manipulation, except by physician.
penicillin, nafcillin or cephalosporin if *S aureus*	Clindamycin, macrolide (but some group A streptococci are resistant); vancomycin if MRSA	10 d	Treat promptly.
vancomycin if MRSA; nafcillin or oxacillin penicillin + clindamycin	cefazolin; if MRSA, then linezolid or daptomycin cephalosporin or vancomycin + clindamycin	10-14 d	May occur in males. Desquamation occurs. Clindamycin added to halt exotoxin production. Consider IVIG.
For staphylococci/ streptococci: nafcillin, cephalosporin For polymicrobial: piperacillin/tazobactam ertapenem, imipenem, meropenem, ampicillin/sulbactam Use or add vancomycin if concern for MRSA	staphylococci/ streptococci: clindamycin, vancomycin polymicrobial: tigecycline* clindamycin + ciprofloxacin or levofloxacin; linezolid or daptomycin if MRSA	clinically determined	Drainage. Exact program depends on bacteria isolated. If abdominal source, use anaerobic agent.
For staphylococci/ streptococci: nafcillin, cephalosporin For polymicrobial: piperacillin/tazobactam ertapenem, imipenem, meropenem, ampicillin/sulbactam Use or add vancomycin if concern for MRSA	staphylococci/ streptococci: clindamycin, vancomycin polymicrobial: tigecycline* clindamycin + ciprofloxacin or levofloxacin; linezolid or daptomycin if MRSA	clinically determined	Debridement, drainage Check tetanus immune status.

*Effective for polymicrobial infections, including MRSA, but not for *Pseudomonas* and less effective for *Proteus* sp.

continued on next page

13

Skin and Soft-Tissue Infections *(continued)*

Location	Primary Diagnosis	Secondary Diagnosis/ Contributing Factors	Pathogens
Skin *(continued)*	burns	local	colonization common with *Streptococcus* species, *S aureus*, coliforms *Pseudomonas* herpes simplex
		sepsis	*S pyogenes* *S aureus*
			Serratia *Providencia* *Pseudomonas*
			Candida
	decubitus ulcers		*S aureus* group A streptococci anaerobes coliforms *Pseudomonas*
	necrotic ulcer (anthrax)		*B anthracis*

Empiric Choices	Alternatives	Duration	Other Measures/ Comments
topical silver sulfadiazine, mafenide, silver nitrate nitrofurazone		clinically determined	It is suggested to follow wound by punch biopsy. Use systemic antibiotics if colonies greater than 10^5/g tissue, or septic course.
penicillin for *S pyogenes*; nafcillin for *S aureus*	cephalosporin; vancomycin, linezolid, daptomycin if MRSA	clinically determined	Debridement.
cefepime, ceftazidime, piperacillin, imipenem, meropenem +/- aminoglycoside	ciprofloxacin, levofloxacin, aztreonam + aminoglycoside	clinically determined	Remove all catheters, if possible.
amphotericin B fluconazole	caspofungin	unknown	Remove catheters. Vein extirpation.
ampicillin/sulbactam, ertapenem. If *Pseudomonas* is a concern: piperacillin/ tazobactam, cefepime, imipenem meropenem	ciprofloxacin or levofloxacin + clindamycin or metronidazole, If MRSA, vancomycin, linezolid, daptomycin	clinically determined	Debridement often necessary for cure.
ciprofloxacin doxycycline	levofloxacin ofloxacin or other quinolones	60 days▲	Prophylaxis for subjects exposed to spores. **Not contagious from person to person.**

▲ Treatment: ciprofloxacin, 400 mg IV q 12 h; doxycycline, 100 mg IV q 12 h
▲ Prophylaxis: ciprofloxacin, 500 mg P.O. q 12 h; doxycycline, 100 mg P.O. q 12 h

continued on next page

Skin and Soft-Tissue Infections *(continued)*

Location	Primary Diagnosis	Secondary Diagnosis/ Contributing Factors	Pathogens
Skin *(continued)*	fungal infections	tinea capitis	*Microsporum* *Trichophyton*
		tinea corporis	dermatophytes
		tinea pedis tinea manuum	*Trichophyton* *Epidermophyton*
		tinea cruris	dermatophytes
		candidiasis (moniliasis)	*C albicans*
	viral infections	underlying diseases: lymphoma renal transplant	herpes zoster
	Lyme arthritis (erythema chronicum migrans) migratory arthritis; large joints	infectious agent spread by tick (*Ixodes dammini*); may be immune-mediated	*Borrelia burgdorferi*

Empiric Choices	Alternatives	Duration	Other Measures/ Comments
terbinafine itraconazole fluconazole	griseofulvin	6-8 wk	Topical agents may not be useful.
topical terbinafine miconazole clotrimazole	oral terbinafine ketoconazole fluconazole	2-4 wk	Oral agents for extensive lesions.
as above	as above	as above, but may need treatment for 6-8 wk	Use 'breathable' material or open sandals for feet.
as above	as above	7-14 d	If irritation occurs, change therapy.
topical clotrimazole	topical miconazole, gentian violet oral fluconazole ketoconazole	7-14 d	
famciclovir acyclovir valacyclovir		10-14 d	Early therapy in the immunocompromised may prevent spread, systemic involvement, and post-herpetic pain.
doxycycline 100 mg P.O. q 12 h amoxicillin 500 mg q 8 h	cefuroxime axetil 500 mg P.O. q 8 h	14-21 d 14-21 d	Meningoencephalitis and carditis may occur. Early penicillin therapy may abort arthritis and carditis. Use parenteral penicillin for neurologic lesions. IV ceftriaxone 2-4 g/d has been successful in some trials for late CNS involvement and arthritis.

13

Section 14: Septicemia

Generalized Infection

Septicemia, sepsis, bacteremia. Fever, chills, hypotension, petechiae, purpura. Initially hyperpnea with respiratory alkalosis progressing to metabolic acidosis. Metastatic abscesses.

Location	Predisposing Factors	Contributing Factors	Pathogens
Genitourinary Tract	indwelling catheters, instrumentation	prostatic obstruction, stones	*E coli, Klebsiella, Enterobacter, Serratia, Pseudomonas, Proteus,* enterococci
Gastrointestinal Tract–Biliary	cholangitis	stones surgery malignancy	*E coli* *Klebsiella* *Bacteroides* enterococci
Large Bowel	abscesses diverticula	neoplasia leukemia	streptococci *Pseudomonas* *Bacteroides* gram-negative bacilli
Reproductive System	surgery abortion postpartum	pregnancy neoplasia	*Bacteroides,* group B streptococci, enterococci, *E coli*

Shock, renal failure. Oxygen, fluid replacement, support blood pressure. Obtain blood, urine, and other cultures before starting therapy.

Empiric Choices:

In each of the choices listed, a third-generation cephalosporin may be used *initially* instead of combination therapy (enterococci are resistant).

Empiric Choices	Alternatives	Duration	Other Measures/ Comments
aminoglycoside* or aztreonam or piperacillin or mezlocillin, TMP/SMX or 3rd-generation cephalosporin or ticarcillin/clavulanate ciprofloxacin, ofloxacin cefepime		based on clinical judgment	Remove catheter as soon as possible.
ampicillin/sulbactam or 3rd-generation cephalosporin + metronidazole, piperacillin/tazobactam, aminoglycoside or aztreonam may be added.	ticarcillin/ clavulanate ciprofloxacin	based on clinical judgment	Surgery needed; drain abscess.
clindamycin + aztreonam or an aminoglycoside; piperacillin/tazobactam;** ampicillin/sulbactam,*** cefoxitin,**** cefotetan**** metronidazole + aminoglycoside cefepime + metronidazole	quinolones (used in conjunction with metronidazole)	based on clinical judgment	Remove infected tissue. Use ultrasound or CAT scan to diagnose abscess.
clindamycin or cefoxitin**** or cefotetan**** + aminoglycoside or aztreonam; ampicillin/sulbactam, ticarcillin/clavulanate, piperacillin, mezlocillin or metronidazole + aminoglycoside piperacillin/tazobactam	quinolones† for gram-negative aerobes	based on clinical judgment	Remove infecting material surgically.

* Aminoglycoside refers to gentamicin or tobramycin. Where resistant *Serratia, Pseudomonas,* or indole-positive *Proteus* is suspected, amikacin is usually active.

** An aminoglycoside should be added.

*** Not for *Pseudomonas.*

**** Do not use aztreonam with cefoxitin or cefotetan; cefoxitin and cefotetan not active against *Pseudomonas.*

† Not to be used in pregnant women.

continued on next page

Septicemia *(continued)*

Location	Predisposing Factors	Contributing Factors	Pathogens
Respiratory Tract	tracheostomy, ventilatory apparatus antibiotics	chronic lung disease	*Enterobacter, Klebsiella, Serratia, Pseudomonas, Proteus, E coli*
Skin	burns	leukemia	*Pseudomonas, Providencia Serratia*
Vascular System	intravenous catheters, foreign bodies, surgery	hospitalization	*Enterobacter, Serratia, Candida, S epidermidis,* enterococci *Pseudomonas*
			J K-diphtheroids

Empiric Choices	Alternatives	Duration	Other Measures/ Comments
aminoglycoside or aztreonam + cefoperazone or ceftazidime (if *Pseudomonas*) or 3rd-generation cephalosporin; piperacillin or piperacillin/tazobactam + an aminoglycoside or mezlocillin + an aminoglycoside or aztreonam ofloxacin ciprofloxacin cefepime		based on clinical judgment	Metronidazole failures in aspiration pneumonia. Use anti-anaerobic agents with quinolones for treatment of mixed infections.
cefepime ceftazidime or piperacillin/tazobactam or piperacillin or azlocillin or cefoperazone + aminoglycoside	ciprofloxacin	based on clinical judgment	Use topical sulfa preparation.
3rd-generation cephalosporin or cefepime	aztreonam (for gram-negatives) piperacillin/ tazobactam piperacillin/ tazobactam + an aminoglycoside	based on clinical judgment	Select agent for pathogen. Change IV.
vancomycin			

14

Section 15: Human Immunodeficiency Virus and Acquired Immunodeficiency Syndrome

Gary P. Wormser, MD

Human immunodeficiency virus (HIV) infection is a chronic infection in which helper T cells ($CD4^+$ cells) are gradually depleted and patients become vulnerable to certain opportunistic infections and neoplasms. The $CD4^+$ lymphocyte count is the most informative marker of the patient's risk for morbidity and mortality. Higher plasma viral loads correlate with a faster rate of decline in the number of $CD4^+$ lymphocytes.

The available antiretroviral agents are nucleoside (or nucleotide) and nonnucleoside reverse transcriptase inhibitors (NRTIs and NNRTIs), protease inhibitors (PIs), and one agent that interferes with fusion of HIV to the $CD4^+$ cell membrane. Antiretroviral therapy is most effective in reducing plasma viral load and delaying the emergence of resistant HIV strains when given in a therapeutic combination of at least three drugs and managed by a clinician with expertise in its use. However, therapy does not eradicate HIV, and HIV will become detectable when the drugs are discontinued.

The clinician must balance potential adverse effects with the need for chronic drug treatment. Most of the challenges in the care of HIV-infected patients in the Western world revolve around decisions on how to use antiretroviral therapy most effectively. This field of medical management is highly complex and rapidly evolving; Internet-based sources often provide the most up-to-date information. The US Department of Health and Human Services provides guidelines for the use of antiretroviral agents in specific patient populations on its Web site: http://aidsinfo.nih.gov/guidelines.

Initiation of antiretroviral therapy is typically delayed to reduce toxicity risks and adherence challenges, but therapy should be prescribed before the $CD4^+$ cell count falls below 200 cells/mm^3. Therapy should be offered to all adult patients with $CD4^+$ cell counts of <350 cells/mm^3 (Table 1).

When selecting an antiretroviral regimen, the clinician should consider several factors, including (1) comorbidities; (2) adherence potential; (3) dosing convenience regarding pill burden, dosing frequency, and food and fluid considerations; (4) potential adverse drug effects; (5) potential interactions with other medications; (6) pretreatment $CD4^+$ cell count; (7) sex; and (8) pregnancy potential.

NNRTI-based regimens include one NNRTI plus two NRTIs. PI-based regimens include one PI (often with ritonavir boosting) plus two NRTIs. Both of these regimens are preferred. Triple NRTI-based regimens have been less successful and should not be used as first-line therapy. Monotherapy and dual-nucleoside regimens are not recommended. Lower-than-therapeutic doses of ritonavir are often added to PI-based regimens to boost the blood level of the PI through inhibition of hepatic metabolism.

In adolescents, dosages of medications for HIV infection and opportunistic infections should be determined according to the Tanner stage of puberty rather than age.

Suppression of plasma viremia to below detectable limits is the immediate goal of therapy, with the ultimate objective of immune stabilization or improvement. Viral suppression should be achieved by 16 to 24 weeks. When this is not possible, partial suppression may still help to prevent further immunologic deterioration.

Adequate viral suppression is typically associated with an increase in $CD4^+$ cell count that averages 100 to 150 cells/mm^3 per year until a threshold is reached. A low baseline $CD4^+$ cell count may be associated with less response to therapy. A significant change between two $CD4^+$ cell count determinations (two standard deviations) is an approximately 30% change in absolute count or a 3-point change in $CD4^+$ cell percentage. A significant change in plasma viral load (two standard deviations) is a threefold change or a change of 0.5 log_{10} copies/mL.

A medication adherence rate of >95% is necessary to delay the emergence of drug-resistant strains of HIV. Adverse effects have been reported with almost all antiretroviral drugs and are among the most common reasons for switching or discontinuing therapy and for medication nonadherence. All PIs and NNRTIs are metabolized in the liver by the cytochrome P450 (CYP) system, particularly by the CYP3A4 isoenzyme. Therefore, the list of drugs with possible interactions is extensive and constantly expanding.

Reasons to consider a change in antiretroviral therapy include (1) failure to decrease viral load by >0.5 log_{10} after 8 weeks of therapy; (2) failure to decrease viral load to undetectable levels by 16 to 24 weeks of therapy; (3) repeated detection of HIV after initial suppression; and (4) threefold or greater increase in viral load from nadir levels, not attributable to some factor unrelated to antiretroviral drug efficacy.

HIV drug resistance testing should be performed to assist in selecting active drugs when changing an antiretroviral regimen in cases of virologic failure. Testing should be done while the patient is on the failing regimen or within 4 weeks of its discontinuation. When changing a regimen for virologic failure, consider the treatment history and past and current resistance test results to identify active agents (preferably three or more) to design a new regimen. Therapeutic drug monitoring of PI and NNRTI blood levels may be useful in selected patients.

Table 1: Indications for Initiating Antiretroviral Therapy for the Chronically HIV-1 Infected Patient*

Clinical Category	$CD4^+$ T Cell Count
AIDS-defining illness or severe symptoms**	Any value
Asymptomatic†	<200/mm^3
Asymptomatic	>200/mm^3 but ≤350/mm^3
Asymptomatic	>350/mm^3
Asymptomatic	>350/mm^3

*Panel on Clinical Practices for Treatment of HIV Infection: Guidelines for the Use of Antiretroviral Agents in HIV-1-Infected Adults and Adolescents: April 7, 2005. Available at: http://AIDSinfo.nih.gov. Accessed August 1, 2005.

**AIDS-defining illness per Centers for Disease Control and Prevention, 1993. Severe symptoms include unexplained fever or diarrhea >2-4 weeks, oral candidiasis, or >10% unexplained weight loss.

†Clinical benefit has been demonstrated in controlled trials only for patients with $CD4^+$ T cells <200/mm^3; however, most clinicians would offer therapy at a threshold of <350 cells/mm^3. A collaborative analysis of data from 13 cohort studies from Europe and North America found that lower $CD4^+$ count, higher HIV viral load, injection drug use, and age over 50 years were all predictors of progression to AIDS or death in antiretroviral-naïve patients beginning combination antiretroviral therapy. These data indicate that the prognosis is better for patients who initiate therapy at >200 cells/mm^3, but risk after initiation of therapy does not vary considerably at >200 cells/mm^3.

Plasma HIV RNA	Recommendation
Any value	Treat
Any value	Treat
Any value	Treatment should be offered after full discussion of pros and cons with each patient
≥100,000	Most clinicians recommend deferring therapy, but some will treat
<100,000	Defer therapy

15

Human Immunodeficiency Virus and Acquired Immunodeficiency Syndrome* *(continued)*

Nucleoside Reverse Transcriptase Inhibitors (NRTI)

Agent Dose/Form	Brand Name	Mechanism of Action	Dosing	Dosing Adjustments
abacavir 300 mg tab oral solution: 20 mg/mL	Ziagen	Nucleoside analogue HIV reverse transcrip-tase (RT) inhibitor	Adults: 300 mg b.i.d. with or without food or 600 mg once daily. Children: See package insert for pediatric dosing.	No need for dosage adjustment in renal insufficiency. No dosage recommenda-tion in patients with hepatic impairment.
zidovudine 100 mg cap 300 mg tab syrup: 10 mg/mL IV: 10 mg/mL	Retrovir (ZDV, AZT)	Nucleoside analogue RT inhibitor	Adults: 300 mg b.i.d. or 200 mg t.i.d. with or without food. Children: See package insert for pediatric dosing.	End-stage renal disease 100 mg t.i.d. No dosage recommend-ation in patients with hepatic impairment.

***Because of the potency, potential toxicities, and changing reports of additional reactions and interactions of these drugs, clinicians must review the most recent complete package insert for each drug.**

Adverse Drug Reactions	Drug Interactions: See package insert for complete and most up-to-date listings
Hypersensitivity reaction (symptoms may include fever, rash, nausea, vomiting, malaise, fatigue, loss of appetite, and respiratory symptoms such as sore throat, cough, and shortness of breath) in 5%. Should not restart after hypersensitivity reaction—may be fatal. Lactic acidosis/severe hepatomegaly with steatosis, including fatal cases.	Not significantly metabolized by CYP-450. Alcohol increases abacavir levels 40%; abacavir has no effect on alcohol levels.
Bone marrow suppression: anemia and/or granulocytopenia; gastrointestinal (GI) intolerance, headache, insomnia, asthenia. Lactic acidosis/severe hepatomegaly with steatosis, including fatal cases. Some patients require erythropoietin to support hematopoiesis.	Ganciclovir, alpha-interferon, 5-flucytosine, and vincristine may increase hematologic effects. Methadone increases ZDV AUC by 43%; ribavirin inhibits phosphorylation of ZDV; probenecid increases blood levels by 100%; potential antagonism of antiretroviral effect by stavudine.

continued on next page

Human Immunodeficiency Virus and Acquired Immunodeficiency Syndrome* *(continued)*

Nucleoside Reverse Transcriptase Inhibitors (NRTI) *(continued)*

Agent Dose/Form	Brand Name	Mechanism of Action	Dosing	Dosing Adjustments
didanosine 25, 50, 100, 150, 200 mg buffered tabs 100, 167, 250 mg buffered powder for solution 125, 200, 250, 400 mg delayed-release capsules	Videx (ddI) Videx EC	Nucleoside analogue RT inhibitor	Adults ≥60 kg: 400 mg once daily (buffered tablet or EC capsule) or 200 mg b.i.d. (buffered tablets) or 250 mg b.i.d. (buffered powder) on an empty stomach. Adults <60 kg: 250 mg daily (buffered tablets or EC capsule) or 125 mg b.i.d. (buffered tablets) or 167 mg b.i.d. (buffered powder) on an empty stomach. Children: See package insert for pediatric dosing.	Dosage adjustment required for renal insufficiency. No dosage recommendation for hepatic impairment. See package insert for complete details.
zalcitabine 0.375 mg tab 0.750 mg tab	Hivid (ddC)	Nucleoside RT inhibitor	0.75 mg q 8 h with or without food	• C_{cr} >40: 0.75 mg q 8 h • C_{cr} 10-40: 0.75 mg q 12 h • C_{cr} <10: 0.75 mg q 24 h No dosage recommendation for hepatic impairment.

***Because of the potency, potential toxicities, and changing reports of additional reactions and interactions of these drugs, clinicians must review the most recent complete package insert for each drug.**

C_{cr} = creatinine clearance

Adverse Drug Reactions	Drug Interactions: See package insert for complete and most up-to-date listings
Pancreatitis, peripheral neuropathy, diarrhea. Lactic acidosis/ severe hepatomegaly with steatosis, including fatal cases. Avoid with stavudine in pregnancy.	Buffered ddI may decrease absorption of atazanavir, indinavir, dapsone, ketoconazole, itraconazole, ciprofloxacin, and tetracyclines (administer 2 h before ddI). Levels increased with tenofovir. Buffered ddI AUC decreased 63% by methadone. Oral ganciclovir increases ddI levels, while ganciclovir levels are reduced; therefore, appropriate doses of the combination of these drugs have not been established. Avoid ribavirin due to an increase in intracellular levels of active metabolite of ddI. Allopurinol increases ddI levels fourfold. Try to avoid other drugs that cause pancreatitis or neuropathy.
Peripheral neuropathy (22% to 35%), stomatitis (13%), rash, and pancreatitis. Lactic acidosis/severe hepatomegaly with steatosis, including fatal cases.	Try to avoid other drugs that cause neuropathy or pancreatitis. Probenecid and cimetidine increase ddC levels. Bioavailability reduced by magnesium-/ aluminum-containing antacids. Avoid use with 3TC due to theoretic risk of antagonism.

continued on next page

Human Immunodeficiency Virus and Acquired Immunodeficiency Syndrome* *(continued)*

Nucleoside Reverse Transcriptase Inhibitors (NRTI) *(continued)*

Agent Dose/Form	Brand Name	Mechanism of Action	Dosing	Dosing Adjustments
stavudine 15, 20, 30, 40 mg caps oral solution: 1 mg/mL	Zerit (d4T)	Nucleoside analogue RT inhibitor	Adults ≥60 kg: 40 mg q 12 h. Adults <60 kg: 30 mg q 12 h with or without food. Children: See package insert for pediatric dosing.	• C_{cr} >50: ≥60 kg: 40 mg q 12 h <60 kg: 30 mg q 12 h • C_{cr} 26-50: ≥60 kg: 12 mg q 12 h <60 kg: 15 mg q 12 h • C_{cr} 10-25: ≥60 kg: 20 mg q 24 h <60 kg: 15 mg q 24 h • Hemodialysis: ≥60 kg: 20 mg q 24 h <60 kg: 15 mg q 24 h No dosage recommendation for hepatic impairment.
lamivudine 150, 300 mg tab oral solution: 10 mg/mL	Epivir (3TC)	Nucleoside analogue RT inhibitor	Tablets- Adults: 300 mg q 24 h or 150 mg q 12 h with or without food. Children: See package insert for pediatric dosing.	• C_{cr} ≥50: 150 mg q 12 h; 300 mg q 24 h • C_{cr} 30-49: 150 mg q 24 h • C_{cr} 15-29: 150 mg x 1, then 100 mg q 24 h • C_{cr} 5-14: 150 mg x 1, then 50 mg q 24 h • C_{cr} <5: 50 mg x 1, then 25 mg q 24 h No dosage recommendation for hepatic impairment.

***Because of the potency, potential toxicities, and changing reports of additional reactions and interactions of these drugs, clinicians must review the most recent complete package insert for each drug.**

C_{cr} = creatinine clearance

Adverse Drug Reactions	Drug Interactions
Peripheral neuropathy; pancreatitis; lipodystrophy; rapidly progressing ascending neuromuscular weakness (rare); hyperlipidemia. Lactic acidosis/severe hepatomegaly with steatosis, including fatal cases (higher incidence with d4T than with other NRTIs).	Avoid use with zidovudine due to potential for drug antagonism; try to avoid other drugs that cause pancreatitis or neuropathy. Avoid didanosine due to increased risk for neuropathy, pancreatitis, and lactic acidosis.
Minimal toxicity; exacerbation of hepatitis B after withdrawal. Lactic acidosis/severe hepatomegaly with steatosis, including fatal cases.	Avoid use of ddC due to theoretic risk of antagonism.

15

continued on next page

Nucleoside Reverse Transcriptase Inhibitors (NRTI) *(continued)*

Agent Dose/Form	Brand Name	Mechanism of Action	Dosing	Dosing Adjustments
emtricitabine 200 mg capsule	Emtriva	Nucleoside RT inhibitor	Adults: 200 mg q 24 h with or without food. Children: See package insert for pediatric dosing.	• C_{cr} ≥50: 200 mg q 24 h • C_{cr} 30-49: 200 mg q 48 h • C_{cr} 15-29: 200 mg q 72 h • C_{cr} <15: 200 mg q 96 h No dosage recommendation for hepatic impairment.
tenofovir 300 mg tablet	Viread	Nucleotide RT inhibitor	Adults: 300 mg q 24 h with or without food. Children: See package insert for pediatric dosing.	• C_{cr} ≥50: 300 mg q 24 h • C_{cr} 30-49: 300 mg q 48 h • C_{cr} <30: Not recommended No dosage recommendation for hepatic impairment.

***Because of the potency, potential toxicities, and changing reports of additional reactions and interactions of these drugs, clinicians must review the most recent complete package insert for each drug.**

C_{cr} = creatinine clearance

Adverse Drug Reactions	**Drug Interactions**
Minimal toxicity; exacerbations of hepatitis B after withdrawal of agent. Lactic acidosis/severe hepatomegaly with steatosis, including fatal cases.	
Asthenia, headache, diarrhea, nausea, vomiting, flatulence, renal insufficiency; exacerbation of hepatitis B after withdrawal of the agent. Lactic acidosis/severe hepatomegaly with steatosis, including fatal cases.	Increases levels of didanosine (40%). Levels increased by lopinavir/ritonavir. Reduces levels of atazanavir; therefore, concomitant administration requires ritonavir boosting.

Protease Inhibitors (PI)

Agent Dose/Form	Brand Name	Mechanism of Action	Dosing	Dosing Adjustments
amprenavir 50 mg gelatin capsules 15 mg/mL oral solution Capsules and oral solution are not bioequivalent on a mg-to-mg basis.	Agenerase (APV)	PI	Adults: 1,400 mg b.i.d. (oral solution) with or without food, but avoid high-fat meal due to decreased absorption. Children: See package insert for pediatric dosing.	Oral solution not recommended in patients with renal or hepatic failure. See package insert for complete details.
fosamprenavir 700 mg tablet	Lexiva	PI (prodrug of amprenavir)	Adults: 1,400 mg q 12 h; 1,400 mg q 24 h with ritonavir 200 mg q 24 h; 700 mg q 12 h with ritonavir 100 mg q 12 h with or without food. Once-daily regimens not recommended for PI-experienced patients. Children: See package insert for pediatric dosing.	No reduction required in renal insufficiency. In hepatic impairment: • Child-Pugh score 5-8, 700 mg b.i.d. • Child-Pugh score 9-12, not recommended Ritonavir boosting should not be used in patients with hepatic impairment.

***Because of the potency, potential toxicities, and changing reports of additional reactions and interactions of these drugs, clinicians must review the most recent complete package insert for each drug.**

Adverse Drug Reactions	Drug Interactions
GI intolerance, nausea, vomiting, diarrhea, rash, oral paresthesias, hyperlipidemia, transaminase elevation, hyperglycemia, fat maldistribution; possible increased bleeding episodes in patients with hemophilia. Drug should be used with caution in patients with sulfonamide allergy.	Many drug interactions due to effects on CYP-450 enzyme system. Space at least 1 h from antacids and buffered didanosine. Amprenavir is formulated with large amounts of vitamin E; avoid supplemental dose of vitamin E. Oral solution contains 55% propylene glycol and is contraindicated in patients taking metronidazole or disulfiram. See package insert for complete listing of all drug interactions.
Skin rash (19%), diarrhea, nausea, vomiting, headache, hyperlipidemia, transaminase elevation, hyperglycemia, fat maldistribution; possible increased bleeding episodes in patients with hemophilia. Drug should be used with caution in patients with sulfonamide allergy.	See amprenavir for effects on CYP-450 enzyme system. When 1,400 mg q 24 h fosamprenavir and ritonavir used with efavirenz, increase ritonavir to 300 mg q 24 h. Coadministration with H_2 blockers decreases levels; therefore, separate times of administration. Coadministration of proton pump inhibitors is expected to decrease amprenavir levels; do not coadminister if possible.

continued on next page

Human Immunodeficiency Virus and Acquired Immunodeficiency Syndrome* *(continued)*

Protease Inhibitors (PI) *(continued)*

Agent Dose/Form	Brand Name	Mechanism of Action	Dosing	Dosing Adjustments
saquinavir 200 mg hard gelatin caps 500 mg tablets	Invirase	PI	Unboosted SQV not recommended. With ritonavir: Adults: ritonavir 100 mg + SQV 1,000 mg b.i.d.; take within 2 h of a meal. Children: See package insert for pediatric dosing.	For both formulations: No adjustments are necessary in renal insufficiency. Exercise caution when administering to patients with hepatic dysfunction.
200 mg soft gelatin caps (refrigerate capsules) Formulations are not bio-equivalent.	Forto-vase	PI		
ritonavir 100 mg cap (refrigerate caps) oral solution: 600 mg/ 7.5 mL (keep oral solution at room temperature)	Norvir	PI	Adults: initiate at 300 mg b.i.d. with food, then increase up to 600 mg b.i.d. by day 14. Children: See package insert for pediatric dosing.	No dose adjustment needed with renal insufficiency. Use caution in hepatic insufficiency. Used at lower doses to boost levels of other protease inhibitors.

***Because of the potency, potential toxicities, and changing reports of additional reactions and interactions of these drugs, clinicians must review the most recent complete package insert for each drug.**

Adverse Drug Reactions	Drug Interactions
GI intolerance, nausea, diarrhea, headache, elevated transaminase enzymes, hyperlipidemia, hyperglycemia, fat maldistribution; possible increased bleeding episodes in patients with hemophilia.	Rifampin should not be used with SQV due to potential for increased liver enzymes. Many drug interactions due to effects on CYP-450 enzyme system; see package insert for most up-to-date listing. Efavirenz not recommended due to decreased SQV levels.
GI intolerance, nausea, vomiting, diarrhea, paresthesias (circumoral and extremities), hyperlipidemia (especially hypertriglyceridemia), hepatitis, asthenia, taste perversion, hyperglycemia, fat maldistribution; possible increased bleeding episodes in patients with hemophilia.	Many drug interactions due to effects on CYP-450 enzyme system; see package insert for most up-to-date listing.

continued on next page

Protease Inhibitors (PI) *(continued)*

Agent Dose/Form	Brand Name	Mechanism of Action	Dosing	Dosing Adjustments
indinavir 200, 333, 400 mg caps	Crixivan	PI	Adults: 800 mg q 8 h on an empty stomach or with skim milk or a low-fat meal; 800 mg b.i.d. with ritonavir 100 or 200 mg b.i.d. Must drink 1.5 L of fluid/d for adequate hydration. Children: See package insert for pediatric dosing.	No dose adjustment needed with renal insufficiency. For mild to moderate hepatic insufficiency due to cirrhosis, 600 mg q 8 h. 800 mg t.i.d. dosage was associated with markedly lower levels in pregnancy, raising concerns about appropriate dosing in this setting.
atazanavir 100, 150, 200 mg capsules	Reyataz	PI	Adults: 400 mg q 24 h; 300 mg q 24 h combined with ritonavir 100 mg q 24 h. Use this regimen in patients experienced with PIs or if coadministering efavirenz or tenofovir. Take with food to increase levels. Children: See package insert for pediatric dosing.	No adjustment in renal failure. In hepatic impairment: • Child-Pugh class 7-9, 300 mg q.d. • Child-Pugh class >9, not recommended

***Because of the potency, potential toxicities, and changing reports of additional reactions and interactions of these drugs, clinicians must review the most recent complete package insert for each drug.**

Adverse Drug Reactions	Drug Interactions
Nephrolithiasis, GI intolerance, nausea, indirect hyperbilirubinemia, hyperlipidemia, headache, asthenia, blurred vision, dizziness, rash, metallic taste, thrombocytopenia, alopecia, hemolytic anemia, hyperglycemia, fat maldistribution; possible increased bleeding episodes in patients with hemophilia.	Many drug interactions due to effects on CYP-450 enzyme system. Efavirenz decreases levels; when used with efavirenz, increase to 1,000 mg q 8 h or boost with ritonavir. When used with delavirdine, decrease dose to 600 mg q 8 h. Refer to package insert for most up-to-date listings.
Hyperglycemia; fat maldistribution; indirect hyperbilirubinemia; possible increased bleeding episodes in patients with hemophilia. Prolonged PR interval—some patients experienced asymptomatic 1st-degree AV block. Use with caution in patients with underlying conduction defects or on concomitant medications that can cause PR prolongation.	Acid-lowering drugs interfere with absorption; for H_2-receptor antagonists, separate dosing by 12 h; do not coadminister proton pump inhibitors. Levels decreased by efavirenz, tenofovir, didanosine. Many drug interactions due to effects on CYP-450 enzyme system; see package insert for most up-to-date listings.

continued on next page

Protease Inhibitors (PI) *(continued)*

Agent Dose/Form	Brand Name	Mechanism of Action	Dosing	Dosing Adjustments
nelfinavir 250, 625 mg tab oral powder: 50 mg/g	Viracept	PI	Adults: 1,250 mg b.i.d. or 750 mg t.i.d.; take with food. Children: See package insert for pediatric dosing.	No dose adjustment in renal insufficiency. Use with caution in hepatic failure. In pregnancy, adequate levels are achieved only by giving 1,250 mg b.i.d.
lopinavir/ ritonavir capsules 133.3 mg lopinavir/ 33.3 mg ritonavir oral solution: 80 mg lopinavir/ 20 mg ritonavir per mL Note: oral solution contains 42% alcohol.	Kaletra	PI (ritonavir has little antiretroviral effect at this dose; it inhibits lopinavir's metabolism by CYP3A)	Adults: 3 capsules (400 mg lopinavir and 100 mg ritonavir) b.i.d. or 5 mL oral solution b.i.d.; take with food Once-daily dosing with 800 mg/200 mg is acceptable in treatment-naïve patients not on efavirenz, nevirapine, amprenavir, fosamprenavir, or nelfinavir. Children: See package insert for pediatric dosing.	No dosage adjustment needed for renal insufficiency. Use with caution in patients with hepatic impairment. Increase dose when used with efavirenz or nevirapine to 533/133 mg b.i.d. Further study is needed to evaluate the significance of reduced lopinavir levels during the 3rd trimester of pregnancy.

***Because of the potency, potential toxicities, and changing reports of additional reactions and interactions of these drugs, clinicians must review the most recent complete package insert for each drug.**

Adverse Drug Reactions	Drug Interactions
Diarrhea, hyperlipidemia, hyperglycemia, fat maldistribution, serum transaminase elevation; possible increased bleeding episodes in patients with hemophilia.	Many drug interactions due to effects on CYP-450 enzyme system; see package insert for most up-to-date listings.
GI intolerance, nausea, vomiting, diarrhea, asthenia, hyperlipidemia (especially hypertriglyceridemia), elevated serum transaminases, hyper-glycemia, fat maldistribution; possible increased bleeding episodes in patients with hemophilia.	Many drug interactions due to effects on CYP-450 enzyme system; see package insert for most up-to-date listing. Solution contains alcohol: avoid with metronidazole and disulfiram.

Nonnucleoside Reverse Transcriptase Inhibitors (NNRTI)

Agent Dose/Form	Brand Name	Mechanism of Action	Dosing	Dosing Adjustments
tipranavir 250 mg capsules (refrigerate)	Aptivus	PI	Adults: 500 mg b.i.d in conjunction with ritonavir 200 mg b.i.d., with food. Children: See package insert for pediatric dosing.	No dosage adjustment expected for renal insufficiency. No dosage adjustment required for mild hepatic impairment (Child-Pugh A). For more severe hepatic impairment, no information is available, and drug should not be used.
nevirapine 200 mg tab oral suspension: 50 mg/5 mL	Viramune	HIV RT inhibitor	Adults: 200 mg q.d. for first 14 d, then 200 mg b.i.d.; take with or without food. Children: See package insert for pediatric dosing.	No adjustment in renal insufficiency; use with caution in hepatic insufficiency.
delavirdine 100, 200 mg tab	Rescriptor	HIV RT inhibitor	Adults: 400 mg t.i.d. with or without food. Children: See package insert for pediatric dosing.	No adjustment in renal insufficiency. Use with caution in hepatic insufficiency.

***Because of the potency, potential toxicities, and changing reports of additional reactions and interactions of these drugs, clinicians must review the most recent complete package insert for each drug.**

Adverse Drug Reactions	Drug Interactions
Hepatic impairment; monitor liver function tests and use with caution in patients with elevated transaminases, chronic hepatitis B or C, or underlying hepatic impairment. Rash; hyperglycemia; fat maldistribution; hyperlipidemia; possible increased bleeding episodes in patients with hemophilia. Use with caution in patients with sulfonamide allergies.	Many drug interactions due to effects on CYP-450 enzyme system; see package insert for most up-to-date listing. Separate in time from administration of aluminum- or magnesium-based antacids due to decreased absorption of tipranavir. Separate in time from administration of didanosine by at least 2 h. Reduce dose of rifabutin by 75%. Capsule contains alcohol; avoid disulfiram and metronidazole.
Rash, including Stevens-Johnson syndrome. Symptomatic hepatitis, including fatal hepatic necrosis; likelihood of this complication is increased in women with CD4$^+$ T-cell counts >250 cells/mm^3 and in men with counts >400 cells/mm^3.	May lower plasma concentrations of other drugs that are extensively metabolized by CYP-3A. Rifampin/rifabutin used only if clearly indicated and with careful monitoring. May decrease concentration of protease inhibitors. May decrease concentration of oral contraceptives. Refer to package insert for complete details.
Rash, pruritus, headache, nausea, increased ALT and AST.	Antacids, H_2-receptor antagonists, and ddI decrease absorption. Metabolized by cytochrome P-450, with many potential drug interactions; see package insert for most up-to-date listing. Increases concentrations of many PIs; coadministration of amprenavir or fosamprenavir not recommended. Decreased levels of delavirdine with phenytoin, phenobarbital, carbamazepine, rifabutin, and rifampin. Rifampin and rifabutin not recommended.

continued on next page

Human Immunodeficiency Virus and Acquired Immunodeficiency Syndrome* *(continued)*

Nonnucleoside Reverse Transcriptase Inhibitors (NNRTI) *(continued)*

Agent Dose/Form	Brand Name	Mechanism of Action	Dosing	Dosing Adjustments
efavirenz 50 mg, 100 mg, 200 mg caps 600 mg tablets	Sustiva	HIV RT inhibitor	Adults: 600 mg q.d. Take at bedtime on an empty stomach. High-fat meals may increase absorption and should be avoided. Children: See package insert for pediatric dosing.	No adjustment in renal insufficiency; use with caution in hepatic insufficiency.

***Because of the potency, potential toxicities, and changing reports of additional reactions and interactions of these drugs, clinicians must review the most recent complete package insert for each drug.**

Adverse Drug Reactions	Drug Interactions
Rash–most mild/moderate that resolves without change in treatment; more common in children. CNS symptoms (dizziness, impaired concentration, somnolence, insomnia, abnormal dreams, hallucinations) in 50% of patients; symptoms improve on therapy. Teratogenic in monkeys. Avoid in pregnancy. False-positive cannabinoid test; increased transaminase levels.	Metabolized by cytochrome P-450, with many potential drug interactions; see package insert for most up-to-date listing. Decreased levels of certain PIs require dosage or regimen modification.

15

Fusion Inhibitors

Agent Dose/Form	Brand Name	Mechanism of Action	Dosing	Dosing Adjustments
enfuvirtide 90 mg SQ injection	Fuzeon	Inhibits fusion of HIV-1 with $CD4^+$ cells	Adults: 90 mg (1 mL) SQ q 12 h Children: See package insert for pediatric dosing. Rotate injection sites with each dose.	No dosage adjustment for renal insufficiency. No dosage recommendation for hepatic impairment.

Combination Agents

Agent Dose/Form	Brand Name	Mechanism of Action	Dosing	Dosing Adjustments
abacavir 300 mg/ zidovudine 300 mg/ lamivudine 150 mg tablet	Trizivir	Nucleoside analogue RT inhibitor	Adults: 1 tab b.i.d. with or without food. Children: See package insert for pediatric dosing.	Not recommended if C_{cr} <50 mL/min.
zidovudine 300 mg/ lamivudine 150 mg tablet	Combivir	Nucleoside analogue RT inhibitor	Adults: 1 tab b.i.d. with or without food. Children: See package insert for pediatric dosing.	Not recommended if C_{cr} <50 mL/min.
abacavir 600 mg/ lamivudine 300 mg tablet	Epzicom	Nucleoside analogue RT inhibitor	Adults: 1 tab daily with or without food. Children: See package insert for pediatric dosing.	Not recommended if C_{cr} <50 mL/min.
emtricitabine 200 mg/ tenofovir 300 mg tablet	Truvada	RT inhibitor	Adults: 1 tab once daily with or without food. Children: See package insert for pediatric dosing.	C_{cr} 30-49: 1 tablet q 48 h. Not recommended if C_{cr} <30 mL/min.

***Because of the potency, potential toxicities, and changing reports of additional reactions and interactions of these drugs, clinicians must review the most recent complete package insert for each drug.**

C_{cr} = creatinine clearance

Fusion Inhibitors *(continued)*

Adverse Drug Reactions	Drug Interactions
Local injection reactions (erythema, induration, nodules,cysts). Increased risk of bacterial pneumonia. Hypersensitivity reaction (<1%)—symptoms may include rash, fever, nausea, vomiting, chills, rigors, hypotension, or elevated serum transaminases; rechallenge is not recommended.	No effect on CYP-450 system.

Combination Agents *(continued)*

Adverse Drug Reactions	Drug Interactions
See abacavir, zidovudine, and lamivudine for details.	See abacavir, zidovudine, and lamivudine.
See zidovudine and lamivudine.	See zidovudine and lamivudine.
See abacavir and lamivudine.	See abacavir and lamivudine.
See emtricitabine and tenofovir.	See emtricitabine and tenofovir.

15

Section 16: Dosages, Interactions, Toxicity

Dosage of Antibiotics*in the Treatment of Serious Infections in Adults and Older Children

Antibiotic	Daily Dose (ranges)*	Usual Interval Between Doses (in hours)*	Average Concentration (µg/mL) Needed to Inhibit Organism: Gram-positive	Average Concentration (µg/mL) Needed to Inhibit Organism: Gram-negative
amikacin	15 mg/kg	8		1-16
azithromycin	500 mg day 1, then 250 mg** 500 mg q.d. x 3 d 1 g, single dose 2 g, single dose	24***		
aztreonam	8 g	8-12	not effective	0.5-8
amoxicillin/ clavulanate (single daily dose)	250 mg/125 mg 500 mg/125 mg 500 mg/125 mg 875 mg/125 mg	8 8 12 12	≤4-2	*H influenzae* ≤4-2
amoxicillin/ clavulanate XR	4,000 mg	12		
ampicillin	12 g	4	0.05-0.5	1-10
ampicillin/sulb.	6-12 g	6	0.5-2.0	2-4
carbenicillin	24-40 g	6	0.1-1.0	1-150
cefamandole	6-12 g	4-6	0.5-1.0	1-16
cefazolin	4-8 g	8	0.05-1.0	1-12
cefdinir	600 mg children: 14 mg/kg	24 24		
cefditoren	800 mg	12		not established
cefepime	1-4 g or 6 g†	12 or 8†	0.5-4	0.05-8
cefixime	400 mg	24	0.25▲	0.25-4
cefonicid	1-2 g	12-24	4	4-8
cefoperazone	2-6 g	8-12	1-2	2-8
ceforanide	0.5-1.0 g	12	2-4	4-16
cefotaxime	6-8 g	6-8	1	0.5-1.0

* Dosage intervals based on normal renal function.
** May be administered IV or P.O. for community-acquired pneumonia.
*** Pediatric dosage: 10 mg/kg, then 5 mg/kg q.d.
† For febrile neutropenia.
▲ Except for *S aureus*.

Antibiotic	Total Daily Dose*	Usual Interval Between Doses (in hours)*	Average Concentration (μg/mL) Needed to Inhibit Organism	
			Gram-positive	Gram-negative
cefotetan	1.5-6 g	12	4-16	1-16
cefoxitin	6-12 g	4-8	1-3	1-16
ceftazidime	6 g	8	1-4	0.5-8.0
ceftibuten	400 mg	24		
ceftizoxime	8-12 g	8	1-2	0.5-8.0
ceftriaxone	1-4 g	12-24	1-2	0.5-8.0
cefuroxime	4.5 g	8	1-2	1-16
cefuroxime axetil	250-1,000 mg	12	0.3-2.0	2-4
cephalothin	6-12 g	4	0.05-1.0	1-16
cephapirin	6-12 g	4-6	0.05-1.0	1-16
chloramphenicol	50-100 mg/kg	6	0.5-2.0	1-10
ciprofloxacin**	500-1,500 mg	12	1-2	0.5
clarithromycin	500-1,000 mg	12	0.03-0.5	0.03-4
clindamycin	2-3 g	6	0.02-1.5	anaerobes only
colistimethate	5 mg/kg	6-8	0.5-2.0	
daptomycin	4 mg/kg	24	0.25-4	not active
dirithromycin	500 mg	24		
ertapenem	1 g	24	0.25	0.06
erythromycin	2-4 g	6	0.05-1.0	
gatifloxacin	400 mg	24	0.5-1.0	1-2
gentamicin	3-6 mg/kg	8		1-5
imipenem/ cilastatin	2 g	6	0.12-4	0.6-4
kanamycin	15 mg/kg	8-12		1-10
levofloxacin	750 mg	24	1-2	0.5-1.0
lincomycin	4-8 g	6	0.5-1.0	
linezolid	1.2 g	12	0.25-4	

*Dosage intervals based on normal renal function.
**Not indicated for children <18 years of age.

continued on next page

Dosage of Antibiotics* in the Treatment of Serious Infections in Adults and Older Children *(continued)*

Antibiotic	Total Daily Dose*	Usual Interval Between Doses (in hours)*	Average Concentration (µg/mL) Needed to Inhibit Organism: Gram-positive	Gram-negative
loracarbef	400-800 mg	12	1-2	0.25-2
meropenem	3 g	8	0.12-4	0.5-4
metronidazole	3 g	8	0.8-4 (anaerobes only)	0.8-4 (anaerobes only)
mezlocillin	12-18 g	4-6	1**	5-10
moxifloxacin	400 mg	24	0.25-0.5	0.5
nafcillin or oxacillin	8-12 g	4-6	0.1-0.3	
ofloxacin	400-800 mg	12	1	0.5
penicillin G	10-24x10^6 mU	4	0.05-0.5	
piperacillin	12-18 g	4-6	1**	5-10; 2-4 for *Pseudomonas*
piperacillin/ tazobactam	13.5 g 20.25 g	6, 8 4	1-4/4	2-8/4
polymyxin B	2.5 mg/kg	6-8		0.5-2.0
quinupristin/ dalfopristin	7.5 mg/kg	8-12	0.5-2	–
tetracycline	2 g	6	0.5-1.0	0.5-3.0
ticarcillin	12-18 g	4	0.1-1.0	1-100
ticarcillin/ clavulanate	12.4-18.6 g	4-6	2-4/2	4-8/2
tigecycline	100 mg	12▲	0.25	2 4 (for anaerobes)
tobramycin	3-6 mg/kg	8	1-6	
trovafloxacin†	200 or 300 mg	24	≤2	≤2
vancomycin	2 g	6	0.5-0.6	

* Dosage intervals based on normal renal function.
** Nonpenicillinase-producing *S aureus.*
▲ Initial dose is 100 mg x 1.
† Serious to fatal liver damage has occurred, so safer alternative antimicrobial therapy is recommended, when available.

Antimicrobial Drug Interactions

Antibiotic/ Antimicrobial*	Interacting Drug	Unwanted Effect	Probable Mode of Action
aminoglycosides	cephalosporin: reported with cephalothin	nephrotoxic	unknown
	curariform neuro-muscular blockers	neuromuscular paralysis	Both exert additive effect.
	cimetidine ranitidine	affects nerve junction in vitro	
	ethacrynic acid, furosemide	eighth-nerve toxicity	additive effect
	methoxyflurane	kidney damage	unknown
	β-lactam antibiotics: penicillins cephalosporins	Inactivate each other. Decreased aminoglycoside activity important when drugs mixed	Binding to charged groups.
chloramphenicol IV	alcohol	disulfiramlike reaction (slight)	Chloramphenicol inhibits metabolism of alcohol.
	hypoglycemics	increased tendency to hypoglycemia	Chloramphenicol inhibits drug detoxification.
	oral anticoagulants	increased anti-coagulant action	Chloramphenicol inhibits drug detoxification.
	phenytoin	tendency to greater toxicity from phenytoin	Chloramphenicol inhibits hepatic microsomal enzymes.
lincomycin or clindamycin	kaolin-pectin	decreased anti-biotic effect	Interference with gastrointestinal absorption of lincomycin.

*For complete prescribing information, especially dosage differentiation, adverse reactions, warnings, and precautions, see appropriate package inserts.

continued on next page

Antimicrobial Drug Interactions *(continued)*

Antibiotic/ Antimicrobial*	Interacting Drug	Unwanted Effect	Probable Mode of Action
isoniazid (INH)	alcohol	greater tendency to hepatitis; decreased INH action	Unknown, enhanced INH metabolism by chronic alcohol intake.
	antacids	decreased INH effects	Interference with INH absorption in gut.
	disulfiram	psychosis; neurologic disorders	Disturbance in metabolism of catecholamines.
	phenytoin	enhanced potential for phenytoin toxicity	Isoniazid inhibits detoxification by microsomes.
linezolid	adrenergic and serotonergic agents, food with high tyramine content	raise blood pressure	reversible inhibitor of monoamine oxidase.
polymyxin	aminoglycosides	kidney damage	Both drugs are nephrotic, giving additive effects.
	curariform agents	neuromuscular paralysis	Both drugs are neuromuscular blockers, giving additive effects.

*See package insert for other contraindications and drug interactions.

Antibiotic/ Antimicrobial*	Interacting Drug	Unwanted Effect	Probable Mode of Action
rifampin	oral anticoagulants	less anticoagulant action	Detoxification enzymes induced by rifampin.
	oral contraceptives	greater pregnancy risk	Estrogen breakdown induced by rifampin.
	probenecid	rifampin toxicity increased	Disturbance of hepatic metabolism of rifampin.
	theophylline ketoconazole chloramphenicol cyclosporine	decreases serum levels	
	corticosteroids	decreases steroid effect	
	quinidine, digoxin	decreases serum levels	Hepatic metabolism.
sulfonamides –especially long-lasting types –including TMP/SMX	oral anticoagulants	enhanced action of anticoagulant	Displacement of anticoagulant from protein binding site.
	oral hypoglycemics	increased hypoglycemia	Unknown; sulfonamides and sulfonylureas have structural similarities.
	methotrexate	neutropenia	unknown
erythromycin*	theophylline cisapride** astemizole** terfenadine**	increases theophylline hexo-barbital, phenytoin cyclosporine, and carbamazepine levels; can cause ventricular arrhythmias	unknown Acts on cytochrome P-450 system

* See package insert for other contraindications and drug interactions.
** Contraindicated. Withdrawn from U.S. market.

continued on next page

16

Dosages, Interactions, Toxicity *(continued)*

Antimicrobial Drug Interactions *(continued)*

Antibiotic/ Antimicrobial*	Interacting Drug	Unwanted Effect	Probable Mode of Action
clarithromycin erythromycin	cisapride** terfenadine** astemizole**	can cause ventricular arrhythmias	Acts on cytochrome P-450 system
azithromycin	aluminum- and magnesium-containing antacids	decreases azithromycin serum levels	
dirithromycin***	cisapride, terfenadine, astemizole	can cause ventricular arrhythmias	Acts on cytochrome P-450 system
telithromycin	itraconazole	↑ C_{max} and AUC of telithromycin	Cytochrome P-450 system 3A4
	ketoconazole	↑ C_{max} and AUC of telithromycin	Cytochrome P-450 system 3A4
	cisapride	↑ in QTc interval	Cytochrome P-450 system 3A4
	pimozide	↑ in pimozide† levels	Cytochrome P-450 system 3A4
	simvastatin	↑ in simvastatin levels	Cytochrome P-450 system 3A4
	midazolam	↑ in AUC of midazolam	Cytochrome P-450 system 3A4
	metoprolol	↑ in C_{max} and AUC of metoprolol	Cytochrome P-450 system 2D6
	digoxin	↑ in digoxin levels but no effect on ECG parameters	

* See package insert for other contraindications and drug interactions.

** Contraindicated. Withdrawn from U.S. market.

*** May interact with terfenadine, cisapride, or astemizole and should not be used together.

† There are no studies looking at the interaction between telithromycin and pimozide, but there is a potential risk of increased pimozide plasma levels by inhibition of CYP- 3A4 pathways by telithromycin as with macrolides.

Antibiotic/ Antimicrobial*	Interacting Drug	Unwanted Effect	Probable Mode of Action
ketoconazole* itraconazole† fluconazole▲	astemizole** terfenadine** cisapride** cyclosporine oral sulfonylureas phenytoin rifampin theophylline warfarin	increase astemizole levels, can cause ventricular arrhythmias can cause ventricular arrhythmias, increases cyclosporine levels may interact with HIV protease inhibitors	Acts on cytochrome P-450 system Acts on cytochrome P-450 system
tetracyclines	oral antacids; calcium-rich foods	decreased antimicrobial effect	Tetracycline chelates divalent ions; leads to decreased absorption of both.
	barbiturates	doxycycline loses effect	Barbiturate-induced hepatic breakdown of doxycycline.
	carbamazepine	doxycycline loses effect	Carbamazepine induces hepatic breakdown of doxycycline.
	oral iron preparations	decreased tetracycline action	Tetracycline chelates divalent ions; leads to decreased absorption of both.
	methoxyflurane	kidney damage	unknown

* See package insert for other contraindications and drug interactions.
** Contraindicated. Withdrawn from U.S. market.
† See page 101 and package insert for numerous interacting drugs.
▲ Fluconazole contraindicated with cisapride and terfenadine.

continued on next page

Dosages, Interactions, Toxicity *(continued)*

Antimicrobial Drug Interactions *(continued)*

Antibiotic/ Antimicrobial*	Interacting Drug	Unwanted Effect	Probable Mode of Action
quinolones	magnesium/ aluminum antacids	decreases quinolone absorption	chelation
	NSAIDs	CNS stimulation	decrease metabolism
		increases:	Metabolites may decrease metabolism.
	theophylline†	• theophylline levels	
	caffeine**	• CNS toxicity	
	warfarin**†	• prothrombin time	
	cyclosporine†	• cyclosporine levels**	
	oral hypoglycemic***	hyperglycemic or hypoglycemic	

* See package insert for other contraindications and drug interactions.

** Not reported with ofloxacin.

*** This effect has been reported with gatifloxacin but is uncommon; may occur more often in the elderly or in patients with renal failure.

† Not reported with trovafloxacin, but serious to fatal liver damage has occurred with trovafloxacin, so safer alternative antimicrobial therapy is recommended, when available.

Toxicity of Antimicrobial Agents

Agent	Mechanism	Signs
hematologic: chloramphenicol	inhibit protein synthesis damage stem cell	reversible anemia leukopenia aplastic anemia
sulfonamide	G6PD deficiency	hemolytic anemia
carbenicillin* ticarcillin* piperacillin mezlocillin ticarcillin/clavulanate piperacillin/tazobactam	platelet aggregation decreased, less with mezlocillin and piperacillin	bleeding
cefamandole cefoperazone cefotetan	vitamin K absorption, decreased inhibition of liver microsomes producing coagulation factors	Increases prothrombin time. Bleeding may be responsive to vitamin K when secondary to hypoprothrombinemia
nervous system: aminoglycosides	binding hair cells of organ of Corti binding vestibular cells competitive neuromuscular blockade	deafness vertigo respiratory paralysis
erythromycin	effect on auditory portion of eighth cranial nerve	after IV use, deafness may be reversible
polymyxin	noncompetitive neuromuscular blockade	respiratory paralysis
penicillin cephalosporin*	cortical stimulation	myoclonic seizures
nalidixic acid	?	peripheral neuritis
metronidazole	?	peripheral neuritis, convulsions

*With high serum levels associated with renal insufficiency.

continued on next page

16

Toxicity of Antimicrobial Agents *(continued)*

Agent	Mechanism	Signs
gastrointestinal: rifampin isoniazid tetracycline	liver cell damage	hepatitis
neomycin	villus damage	malabsorption
clindamycin lincomycin ampicillin and cephalosporin most antibiotics	stool overgrowth with *Clostridium difficile*	diarrhea pseudomembranous colitis
renal: amphotericin B	tubular damage bone marrow depression	azotemia, alkaline urine, pancytopenia
penicillins, methicillin most common	interstitial nephritis	fever, eosinophilia, azotemia, eosinophiluria
cephaloridine	tubular damage	azotemia
aminoglycoside	tubular damage	cylindruria, azotemia
polymyxin	tubular damage	azotemia
muscle involvement: quinupristin/ dalfopristin	unknown	myalgia
daptomycin	myopathy neuropathy	myalgia muscle weakness rise in CPK

Section 17: Dosage Adjustment in Renal and Hepatic Disease

Dosage Adjustment in Renal Disease and Renal Failure

A way to determine dosage adjustment in renal disease and renal failure is to estimate creatinine clearance (C_{cr}) by the following formula:

$$C_{cr} = \frac{(140\text{-age}) \times (\text{wt in kg})}{72 \times \text{serum creatinine}}$$

(Multiply above result by 0.85 in females)

There are two basic methods of adjusting the dose of antibiotics that are predominantly excreted through renal mechanisms. In the first method, the variable frequency regimen (VFR), a loading dose of the antibiotic is given, followed by a 'standard' dose (calculated by mg/kg of body weight) at prolonged time intervals based on the degree of renal dysfunction. In the second, the variable dose regimen (VDR), a loading dose of the drug is followed at set 'standard' time intervals with decreased maintenance doses of the drug based on renal dysfunction.

For aminoglycosides: The appropriate dose of aminoglycoside, gentamicin, or tobramycin, to be used in a patient weighing 70 kg with a serum creatinine of 2 mg/dL for each of the two methods can be:

In the VFR method, a loading dose of 2 mg/kg is given, then a dose of 1 mg/kg is given (8 times the serum creatinine in hours). Thus, in this case the loading dose is 140 mg gentamicin (70 kg x 2 mg/kg) followed by 70 mg every 16 hours.

In the VDR method, the loading dose is the same (2 mg/kg) followed by a maintenance dose calculated as 1 mg/kg of body weight divided by the serum creatinine in the mg/dL (1 mg/kg creatinine) given every 8 hours. The patient with a serum creatinine of 2 would receive 140 mg of gentamicin as a loading dose (70 kg x 2 mg/kg) and then 35 mg every 8 hours (70÷2).

Then refer to the *Reduced Dosage in Renal Failure* Table below.

For netilmicin, the same formula can be used with a special table use to calculate the dose (see package insert).

Consider our 70-kg male patient who is 65 years old and has a serum creatinine of 2 mg/dL. The loading dose is the same as before, 140 mg. The dose given every 8 hours is based on the patient's calculated creatinine clearance. In this case the clearance is calculated to be approximately 35 mL/min. Utilizing the reduced dosage table, the patient would get 50% of the maintenance dose every 8 hours. It is probably wise to use 1.5 mg/kg as the maintenance dose for the first 48 hours, and then to use 1 mg/kg.

In the case of amikacin, similar calculations to those mentioned apply. However, the total daily dose is calculated to be 15 mg/kg. A loading dose of 7.5 mg/kg would be given to our 70-kg patient, or approximately 500-525 mg. The maintenance dose would be calculated, as it was previously, on the basis of the creatinine clearance calculated for age, weight, and serum creatinine.

Serum level monitoring is suggested for more accurate guidance in aminoglycoside dosing because dosage adjustments may lead to suboptimal or toxic levels.

Maximal Dosage Adjustments in Renal Failure*

Degree of Renal Impairment as Determined by Creatinine Clearance (C_{cr}) Values

Drug	C_{cr} Value (mL/min)	Dose (g)
penicillins:		
penicillin G	30-50	no change
ampicillin	30-50	no change
amoxicillin	30-50	no change
ticarcillin	30-50	2
oxacillin**, nafcillin, cloxacillin, dicloxacillin	30-50	no change
cephalosporins:		
cephalothin	10-50	1
cephapirin	10-50	1
cefazolin	10-50	0.5-1.0
cephalexin	10-50	0.25
cephradine	20-50	0.5
cefoxitin	10-50	1-2
cefamandole	10-50	1-2

* All β-lactam antibiotics, whether penicillins or cephalosporins, may produce convulsions in the presence of severe renal failure (Bennet WM, et al: *Ann Intern Med* 1980;93:62).

** Minor change may be necessary.

See Also:

cefonicid–Table 1
ceftazidime–Table 2
cefuroxime–Table 3
cefixime–Table 11
loracarbef–Table 9
clarithromycin–Table 10
cefepime–Table 17
cefotetan–Table 18
daptomycin–Table 25
meropenem–Table 16
cefpodoxime proxetil–Table 19
cefdinir–Table 20
imipenem–Table 21
ertapenem–Table 24
levofloxacin–Table 22
gatifloxacin–Table 23

antivirals:
acyclovir–Tables 4 and 5
ganciclovir–Table 6
valganciclovir–Table 7
famciclovir– Table 12
valacyclovir–Tables 13 and 14
foscarnet–Table 15

antifungals:
fluconazole–Table 8
voriconazole–Table 28

Interval Between Doses (h)	C_{cr} Value (mL/min)	Dose (g)	Interval Between Doses (h)
usual	<10	full loading dose x 1, then 1/2 loading dose	8-10
usual	<10	0.5-1.0	12-24
usual	<10	0.25-0.5	24
4 usual	<10 <10	2 no change	12 no change
4-6 4-6	<10 <10	1 1	8-12 8-12
8-12	<10	0.25-0.5	18-24
6 6	<10 <10	0.25 0.25	12-24 12-24
8-12 6-8	<10 <10	0.5-1.0 0.5-0.75	12-48 8-12

Reduced Dosage in Renal Failure*

	Creatinine Clearance (C_{cr}) mL/min	Percentage of dosage		
		8h	12 h	24 h
gentamicin, tobramycin	80	80	90	–
loading dose: 2 mg/kg	70	75	88	–
maintenance dose:	60	70	85	–
1-1.5 mg/kg	50	65	80	–
	40	55	70	95
	30	45	65	85
amikacin	20	35	50	75
loading dose: 7.5 mg/kg	15	30	40	65
maintenance dose: 5 mg/kg	10	25	35	55

*Blood levels should be obtained whenever renal function is decreased or changing.

Drug Use in Hepatic Failure

trovafloxacin*–Table 26
caspofungin–Table 27

*Serious to fatal liver damage has occurred, so safer alternative antimicrobial therapy is recommended, when available.

Maximal Dosage Adjustments in Renal Failure *(continued)*

Table 1 Dosage Regimen* for Adults With Reduced Renal Function

Drug	C_{cr} Value (mL/min per 1.73 m^2)	Mild to Moderate Infections Dose	Route	Interval Between Doses	Severe Infections Dose	Route	Interval Between Doses
cefonicid	60-79	10 mg/kg	IV or deep IM	24 h	25 mg/kg	IV or deep IM	24 h
	40-59	8 mg/kg		24 h	20 mg/kg		24 h
	20-39	4 mg/kg	↓	24 h	15 mg/kg	↓	24 h
	10-19	4 mg/kg		48 h	15 mg/kg		48 h
	5-9	4 mg/kg		3-5 d	15 mg/kg		3-5 d
	<5	3 mg/kg		3-5 d	4 mg/kg		3-5 d

*Monitor blood levels and adjust dosage accordingly.
Note: No additional dose after dialysis.

Table 2 Dosage Regimen for Patients With Impaired Renal Function

Drug	C_{cr} Value (mL/min)	Dose	Route	Frequency of Dose
ceftazidime	31-50	1 g	IV, IM	q 12 h
	16-30	1 g	IV, IM	q 24 h
	6-15	500 mg	IV, IM	q 24 h
	<5	500 mg	IV, IM	q 48 h
	hemodialysis	1 g	IV, IM	p̄ each dialysis

Table 3 Dosage in Reduced Renal Function

Drug	C_{cr} Value (mL/min)	Dose	Frequency
cefuroxime	>20	750 mg-1.5 g	q 8 h
	10-20	750 mg	q 12 h
	<10	750 mg	q 24 h

Table 4 Dosage Regimen for Patients With Impaired Renal Function

Drug	C_{cr} Value (mL/min per 1.73 m^2)	Percent of Recommended Dose	Dosing Interval
acyclovir IV	>50	100%	8 h
	25-50	100%	12 h
	10-25	100%	24 h
	0-10	50%	24 h

Table 5 Dosage Regimen for Patients With Impaired Renal Function

Drug	Normal Dosage (mg)	C_{cr} Value (mL/min)	Adjusted Dosage	
			Dose (mg)	Dosing Interval
acyclovir oral*	200 q 4 h	>10	200	q 4 h 5x daily
		0-10	200	q 12 h
	400 q 12 h	>10	400	q 12 h
		0-10	200	q 12 h
	800 q 4 h	>25	800	q 4 h 5x daily
		10-25	800	q 8 h
		0-10	800	q 12 h

*For hemodialysis: Administer an additional dose after each dialysis. No supplemental dosing for peritoneal dialysis.

Table 6 Dosage for Adults With Impaired Renal Function

Drug	C_{cr} Value (mL/min)	Dose (mg/kg)	Frequency
ganciclovir intravenous (induction)	≥70	5	q 12 h
	50-69	2.5	q 12 h
	25-49	2.5	q 24 h
	10-24	1.25	q 24 h
	<10	1.25	3 x/week, following hemodialysis
ganciclovir intravenous (maintenance)	≥70	5	q 24 h
	50-69	2.5	q 24 h
	25-49	1.25	q 24 h
	10-24	0.625	q 24 h
	<10	0.625	3 x/week, following hemodialysis
ganciclovir oral	≥70	1,000	t.i.d.
		or	
		500	q 3 h, 6x/day
	50-69	1,500	q.d.
		or	
		500	t.i.d.
	25-49	1,000	q.d.
		or	
		500	b.i.d.
	10-24	500	q.d.
	<10	500	3 x/week, following hemodialysis

Table 7 Dose Modifications for Impaired Renal Function

Drug	C_{cr} Value (mL/min/kg)	Induction Dose	Maintenance/ Prevention Dose
valganciclovir	>60	900 mg b.i.d.	900 mg once daily
	40-59	450 mg b.i.d.	450 mg once daily
	25-39	450 mg once daily	450 mg q 2 days
	10-24	450 mg q 2 days	450 mg twice weekly

Table 8

Drug	C_{cr} Value (mL/min)	% of Recommended Dose
fluconazole*	>50	100%
	≤50	50%
	hemodialysis	1 recommended dose $\bar{p}$ each dialysis

*Give loading dose of 50-400 mg.

Table 9

Drug	C_{cr} Value (mL/min)	Dose	Route	Interval
loracarbef	>50	usual	P.O.	q 12 h
	10-49	usual	P.O.	q 24 h
	or 1/2	P.O.	q 12 h	
	<10	usual	P.O.	q 3-5 days
	hemodialysis	usual	P.O.	after dialysis

Table 10

Drug	C_{cr} Value	Dose	Interval
clarithromycin*	<30	1/2 usual dose same dose	usual interval double interval

*May administer in presence of hepatic impairment without dosage adjustment with normal renal function.

Table 11

Drug	C_{cr} Value (mL/min)	Dose	Route	Dosing Interval
cefixime	>60	adults: 400 mg children: 8 mg/kg	P.O. P.O.	24 h 24 h
	21-60 or hemodialysis	adults: 300 mg	P.O. P.O.	24 h 24 h
	<20 or continuous ambulatory peritoneal dialysis	200 mg	P.O.	24 h

Table 12

Drug	C_{cr} Value (mL/min)	Dose	Frequency
famciclovir	>60	500 mg	q 8 h
	40-59	500 mg	q 12 h
	20-39	500 mg	q 24 h
	<20	250 mg	q 24 h

Maximal Dosage Adjustments in Renal Failure *(continued)*

Table 13

Drug	C_{cr} Value (mL/min)	Dose	Frequency
valacyclovir (for herpes zoster)	>50	1 g	q 8 h
	30-49	1 g	q 12 h
	10-29	1 g	q 24 h
	<10	500 mg	q 24 h
	hemodialysis	1 g	after dialysis
valacyclovir (for genital herpes)	>50	1 g	q 12 h
	30-49	1 g	q 12 h
	10-29	1 g	q 24 h
	<10	500 mg	q 24 h

Table 14

		C_{cr} Value (mL/min)		
Drug	**Normal Dose**	**30-49**	**10-29**	**<10**
valacyclovir (recurrent genital herpes, suppressive therapy)	500 mg q 12 h 1 g q 24 h 500 mg q 24 h	no change no change no change	500 mg q 24 h 500 mg q 24 h 500 mg q 48 h	500 mg q 24 h 500 mg q 24 h 500 mg q 48 h
valacyclovir (genital herpes with HIV, suppressive therapy)	500 mg q 12 h	no change	500 mg q 24 h	500 mg q 24 h
valacyclovir (herpes febrilis [cold sores])*	two 2 g doses q 12 h	two 1 g doses q 12 h	two 500 mg doses q 12 h	one 500 mg dose

*Do not exceed 1 day of treatment.

Table 15 Dosage for Adults With Reduced Renal Function

Drug	Indication	C_{cr} Value (mL/min/kg)	Dose (mg/kg)	Frequency
foscarnet (induction)	To treat: herpes simplex virus (equivalent to 80 mg/kg/day total; normal dose: 40 mg/kg q 12 h)	>1.4	40	q 12 h
		>1.0-1.4	30	q 12 h
		>0.8-1.0	20	q 12 h
		>0.6-0.8	35	q 24 h
		>0.5-0.6	25	q 24 h
		≥0.4-0.5	20	q 24 h
		<0.4	NR*	
	herpes simplex virus (equivalent to 120 mg/kg/day total; normal dose: 40 mg/kg q 8 h)	>1.4	40	q 8 h
		>1.0-1.4	30	q 8 h
		>0.8-1.0	35	q 12 h
		>0.6-0.8	25	q 12 h
		>0.5-0.6	40	q 24 h
		≥0.4-0.5	35	q 24 h
		<0.4	NR*	
	To treat: cytomegalovirus (equivalent to 180 mg/kg/day total; normal dose: 60 mg/kg q 8 h)	>1.4	60	q 8 h
		>1.0-1.4	45	q 8 h
		>0.8-1.0	50	q 12 h
		>0.6-0.8	40	q 12 h
		>0.5-0.6	60	q 24 h
		≥0.4-0.5	50	q 24 h
		<0.4	NR*	
	cytomegalovirus (equivalent to 180 mg/kg/day total; normal dose: 90 mg/kg q 12 h)	>1.4	90	q 12 h
		>1.0-1.4	70	q 12 h
		>0.8-1.0	50	q 12 h
		>0.6-0.8	80	q 24 h
		>0.5-0.6	60	q 24 h
		≥0.4-0.5	50	q 24 h
		<0.4	NR*	
foscarnet (maintenance)	cytomegalovirus (equivalent to 90 mg/kg/day once daily)	>1.4	90	q 24 h
		>1.0-1.4	70	q 24 h
		>0.8-1.0	50	q 24 h
		>0.6-0.8	80	q 48 h
		>0.5-0.6	60	q 48 h
		≥0.4-0.5	50	q 48 h
		<0.4	NR*	
	cytomegalovirus (equivalent to 120 mg/kg/day once daily)	>1.4	120	q 24 h
		>1.0-1.4	90	q 24 h
		>0.8-1.0	65	q 24 h
		>0.6-0.8	105	q 48 h
		>0.5-0.6	80	q 48 h
		≥0.4-0.5	65	q 48 h
		<0.4	NR*	

*Not recommended.

Maximal Dosage Adjustments in Renal Failure *(continued)*

Table 16

Drug	C_{cr} Value (mL/min)	Dose (dependent on infection)	Interval
meropenem	26-50	recommended dose	q 12 h
	10-25	½ recommended dose	q 12 h
	<10	½ recommended dose	q 24 h
	There are inadequate data on usage in patients on hemodialysis and no data for patients on peritoneal dialysis.		

Table 17

Drug	C_{cr} Value (mL/min)	Normal Dose	Normal Dose	Normal Dose	Normal Dose
		Normal Recommended Dosing Schedule			
cefepime	>60	500 mg q 12 h	1 g q 12 h	2 g q 12 h	2 g q 8 h
		Dose Changes Recommended			
	30-60	500 mg q 24 h	1 g q 24 h	2 g q 24 h	2 g q 12 h
	11-29	500 mg q 24 h	500 mg q 24 h	1 g q 24 h	2 g q 24 h
	<10	250 mg q 24 h	250 mg q 24 h	500 mg q 24 h	1 g q 24 h
	Repeat initial dose after dialysis.				

Drug	C_{cr} Value (mL/min)	Dose	Interval Between Doses
aminoglycosides gentamicin, tobramycin, amikacin	See page 251 for table on reduced dosage in renal failure.		
aztreonam	10-30	loading 1-2 g, then ½ usual dose	
	<10 (hemodialysis)	500 mg-2 g initially, then ¼ of above at approp. interval: ⅛ of initial dose after each dialysis	

Drug	C_{cr} Value (mL/min)	Dose	Interval Between Doses
ampicillin/ sulbactam	>30 15-29 5-14	1.5-3.0 g 1.5-3.0 g 1.5-3.0 g	q 6 h q 12 h q 24 h
ciprofloxacin P.O.	>50 30-50 5-29 hemodialysis, peritoneal dialysis	usual dosage 250-500 mg 250-500 mg 250-500 mg	q 12 h q 12 h q 18 h q 24 h after dialysis
IV	>30 5-29	usual dosage 200-400 mg	 q 18-24 h
ofloxacin	 >50 20-50 <20	give normal initial dose, then: usual dosage b.i.d. then usual dosage q.d. 1/2 the usual dosage q.d.	12 h 24 h 24 h 24 h
cefotaxime	<20	50% of dose	usual
piperacillin*	>40 20-40 <20 hemo-dialysis	no change 4 g 4 g 2 g and 1 g after dialysis	usual q 8 h q 12 h q 8 h
piperacillin/ tazobactam	>40 20-40 <20 hemo-dialysis	no change 2.25 g 2.25 g 2.25 g + 0.75 g after each dialysis period	no change q 6 h q 8 h q 8 h
mezlocillin	>30 10-30 <10	no change 3 g 2 g (In dialysis patients, 3 g after dialysis and then 3 g q 12 h)	usual q 8 h q 8 h

*For serious systemic infections; see package insert for dosing for other indications.

17

continued on next page

Table 17 *(continued)*

Drug	C_{cr} Value (mL/min)	Dose	Interval Between Doses
ticarcillin/ clavulanate	>60	3.1 g	q 4 h
	30-60	2 g	q 4 h
	10-30	2 g	q 8 h
	<10	2 g	q 12 h
	<10 with hepatic dysfunction	2 g	q 24 h
	patients on peritoneal dialysis	3.1 g	q 12 h
	patients on hemodialysis	2 g supplemented with 3.1 g after each dialysis	q 12 h
trimethoprim/ sulfamethox-azole	>30	standard dose	q 6 h
	15-30	½ standard dose	q 6 h
	<15	not recommended	

*For serious systemic infections; see package insert for dosing for other indications.

Table 18

Drug	C_{cr} Value (mL/min)	Dose	Frequency
cefotetan	>30	usual recommended dosage*	q 12 h
	10-30	usual recommended dosage*	q 24 h
	<10	usual recommended dosage*	q 48 h
	If patient is being hemodialyzed, give 1/2 dose on days of dialysis and 1/4 dose on days between dialysis.		

*Dose determined by the type and severity of infections and susceptibility of causative organism.

Table 19

Drug	C_{cr} Value (mL/min)	Dose	Interval
cefpodoxime proxetil	<30	usual dose	increase interval q 24 h

Table 20

Drug	C_{cr} Value (mL/min)	Dose
cefdinir	<30	300 mg/d; for hemodialysis patients: 300 mg every other day

Table 21

Drug	C_{cr} Value (mL/min)	Dose	Interval
imipenem*	<70	500 mg	8 h
	<40	500 mg	12 h
	<20	250 mg	12 h

*See package insert for complete information; adjustment depends on usual dose and patient's weight.

Table 22

Drug	C_{cr} Value (mL/min)	Initial Dose	Dose/Interval
levofloxacin*	50-80	No dosage adjustment	
	20-49	500 mg	250 mg q 24 h
	10-19	500 mg	250 mg q 48 h
	hemodialysis	500 mg	250 mg q 48 h
	CAPD	500 mg	250 mg q 48 h

*Dose dependent on infection being treated. See package insert for complete information.

Maximal Dosage Adjustments in Renal Failure *(continued)*

Table 23

Drug	C_{cr} Value (mL/min)	Initial Dose	Subsequent Dose
gatifloxacin	>40	400 mg q.d.	400 mg q.d.
	<40	400 mg q.d.	200 mg q.d.
	hemodialysis	400 mg q.d.	200 mg q.d.
	patients on peritoneal dialysis	400 mg q.d.	200 mg q.d.

Table 24

Drug	C_{cr} Value (mL/min)	Initial Dose	Subsequent Dose
ertapenem	<30	500 mg	500 mg/d
	patients on hemodialysis	500 mg	give supplemental dose of 150 mg after dialysis if initial dose given within 6 h

Table 25

Drug	C_{cr} Value (mL/min)	Initial Dose	Subsequent Dose
daptomycin	<30 hemodialysis* and CAPD	4 mg/kg	q 48 h

*Give daptomycin after dialysis, if possible.

Drug Use in Hepatic Failure

Table 26

Chronic hepatic disease (cirrhosis): This table provides dosing guidelines for patients with mild to moderate cirrhosis (Child-Pugh Class A and B). There are no data in patients with severe cirrhosis (Child-Pugh Class C).

Drug	Indicated Dose (normal hepatic function)	Chronic Hepatic Disease Dose
trovafloxacin*	300 mg IV 200 mg IV or oral	200 mg IV 100 mg IV or oral

*Serious to fatal liver damage has occurred, so safer alternative antimicrobial therapy is recommended, when available.

Table 27

Drug	Indicated Dose	Chronic Hepatic Disease Dose
caspofungin	(normal hepatic function) 70 mg/d, then 50 mg/d	(mild hepatic insufficiency) 70 mg/d then 35 IV

Table 28

Drug	C_{cr} Value (mL/min)	Dose
voriconazole	6 mg/kg IV x 2 doses, then 4 mg/kg q 12 h	6 mg/kg IV x 2 doses, then 2 mg/kg q 12 h

17

Drug Use in Renal Failure

	Drug	Mechanism of Elimination	Toxicity/Comments
no major adjustment needed	amphotericin	nonrenal	Causes tubular damage, decreased renal blood flow, renal tubular acidosis, and hypokalemia.
	azithromycin	primarily liver	
	chloramphenicol	liver (kidney)	
	doxycycline	kidney (liver), GI tract in patients with renal failure	Only tetracycline used in renal failure.
	erythromycin	liver	Rarely, ototoxicity following IV usage.
	isoniazid	liver, kidney	Neurotoxic, hepatotoxic.
	penicillins: cloxacillin dicloxacillin flucloxacillin nafcillin	kidney-tubular plus liver liver	Seizures rare.
	rifampin	liver, GI tract	Interstitial nephritis rare.
	cefaclor	kidney (liver)	
	cefoperazone	liver, kidney	If liver and kidney dysfunction, then adjust dosage.
	ceftriaxone	liver, kidney	If liver and kidney dysfunction, then adjust dosage.
	moxifloxacin	liver, kidney, GI balanced	No dosage adjustment needed.
	linezolid	liver, kidney	No dosage adjustment needed; metabolites may accumulate in serum.
	telithromycin voriconazole*	liver, kidney liver, kidney	No dose adjustment needed when C_{cr} ≥30 mL/min. No dose has been established in severely renally impaired patients with C_{cr} <30 mL/min, including those who need dialysis. No dosage adjustment needed except for IV formulation (because of diluent).
	quinupristin/ dalfopristin	liver, kidney	No dosage adjustment needed.

*The oral dose should be used in patients with renal failure. There are no guidelines for IV use in renal failure patients.

	Drug	Mechanism of Elimination	Toxicity/Comments
minor adjustment needed	lincomycin clindamycin	liver (kidney)	Interval between doses can be increased.
	penicillins: amoxicillin (oral) penicillin V oxacillin	 kidney-tubular kidney (liver)	 Toxicity of the type seen with other penicillins.
	macrolides: clarithromycin dirithromycin	 liver, kidney	For all macrolides, levels may increase in patients with renal disease.
moderate to significant dose adjustment for major renal failure	cephalosporins: cefazolin cephalexin cephapirin cephalothin cephradine cefonicid ceftazidime cefamandole cefoxitin cefotaxime loracarbef aztreonam	 kidney-tubular kidney (liver) kidney	 Interstitial nephritis rarely; use with aminoglycosides possibly adds to toxicity of aminoglycosides. No nephrotoxicity or ototoxicity.
	aminoglycosides: amikacin gentamicin kanamycin netilmicin sisomicin streptomycin tobramycin	 kidney-glomerular	 Nephrotoxic, ototoxic.
	antivirals: acyclovir IV famciclovir valacyclovir ganciclovir	 kidney-glomerular	 Increase levels in renal failure
	ethambutol	kidney	Optic neuritis
	flucytosine	kidney	Neutropenia, thrombocytopenia, GI toxicity

continued on next page

Drug Use in Renal Failure *(continued)*

	Drug	Mechanism of Elimination	Toxicity/Comments
moderate to significant dose adjustment for major renal failure *(continued)*	penicillins: ampicillin ampicillin/sulbactam carbenicillin methicillin penicillin G ticarcillin	kidney-tubular (some liver)	Seizures, interstitial nephritis, sodium overload, hypokalemia
	mezlocillin piperacillin piperacillin/tazobactam	kidney, biliary	(Less sodium load) (Less sodium load) (Less sodium load)
	sulfisoxazole sulfamethoxazole	kidney	Rarely precipitates in tubules.
	trimethoprim	kidney	Questionable decrease in renal function. Hematologic.
	vancomycin	kidney	Ototoxic, nephrotoxicity rare.
	ciprofloxacin	kidney liver	GI, CNS
	ofloxacin	mainly renal	GI, CNS
	norfloxacin	kidney, liver	
	lomefloxacin	mainly renal	GI, CNS
	levofloxacin	mainly renal	GI, CNS
	gatifloxacin	mainly renal	GI

	Drug	Mechanism of Elimination	Toxicity/Comments
avoid in renal impairment if possible	colistimethate*	kidney	Nephrotoxic, peripheral neuropathy, respiratory paralysis
	methenamine mandelate	kidney	Ineffective, acidosis
	nalidixic acid	kidney	Ineffective
	neomycin	kidney	Nephrotoxic-ototoxic
	nitrofurantoin	kidney	Ineffective, peripheral neuritis
	p-aminosalicylic acid (PAS)	kidney, liver	GI toxicity
	polymyxin B* colimycin*	kidney	Nephrotoxic, peripheral neuropathy, respiratory paralysis
	spectinomycin	kidney	Use only single dose.
	tetracyclines: chlortetracycline oxytetracycline tetracyclines HCl minocycline	kidney, liver	Azotemia, nephrotoxic, hepatotoxic

*These agents may need to be used to treat resistant gram-negative infections.

Effect of Dialysis on Antibiotic Blood Levels

	Effect on Blood Levels		Added Dose Given After Dialysis	
Drug	Peritoneal Dialysis	Hemodialysis	Peritoneal Dialysis	Hemodialysis
penicillins:				
penicillin G	slight	yes	variable	yes
ampicillin/ amoxicillin	slight	yes	variable	yes
carbenicillin ticarcillin/	slight	yes	variable	yes
clavulanate	?	yes (?)	?	?
methicillin	no	yes	variable	yes
oxacillin nafcillin cloxacillin	no	no	variable	yes
dicloxacillin piperacillin	slight	yes	variable	yes
piperacillin/ tazobactam	slight	yes	added dose	yes
cephalosporins:				
cephalothin	variable	yes	variable	
cephapirin	variable	yes	variable	yes, usually
cefazolin	variable	yes	variable	0.5-10 g
cefonicid	?	?	no	?
cefuroxime	?	yes	?	yes
cephalexin	variable	yes	variable	
cephradine	variable	yes	variable	
cefoxitin	variable	yes	variable	
cefotetan	unknown	yes	unknown	yes
cefamandole	variable	yes	variable	
cefotaxime	variable	yes	variable	15 mg/kg after dialysis
cefepime	variable	yes	variable	yes
cefoperazone	unknown	yes	unknown	yes
trovafloxacin*	?	no	?	no
linezolid	?	yes↓	?	yes
caspofungin	no	no	no	no

*Serious to fatal liver damage has occurred, so safer alternative antimicrobial therapy is recommended, when available.

Drug	Effect on Blood Levels: Peritoneal Dialysis	Effect on Blood Levels: Hemodialysis	Added Dose Given After Dialysis: Peritoneal Dialysis	Added Dose Given After Dialysis: Hemodialysis
aminoglycosides:				
gentamicin	yes	yes	additional* parenteral dose given with caution if antibiotic added to dialysate. Blood level must be checked.	$\frac{1}{2}$-$\frac{3}{4}$* loading dose for these first three aminoglycosides
tobramycin	yes	yes		
amikacin	yes	yes		
netilmicin	yes	yes		2 mg/kg
antifungals:				
amphotericin	no	no	no change	no change
5-flucytosine	yes	yes	25 mg/kg after dialysis	25 mg/kg after dialysis
fluconazole	?	yes	?	recommended dose
voriconazole	?	no	?	no
lipopeptides:				
daptomycin	no	no	no	no
vancomycin	no	no**	no	no

*Monitor serum levels.
**Vancomycin may be cleared somewhat by high-flux membranes.

17

Section 18: Prophylactic Antibiotics

Advantages

1. Protects healthy susceptible individuals of all ages who are exposed to infections (eg, *N meningitidis* and *M tuberculosis*).

2. Prevents infectious complications after operations in surgically traumatized and potentially contaminated areas (vaginal hysterectomy, biliary tract, colonic surgery, compound fracture, etc).

Prophylaxis in Medical Situations

Bacterial Pathogen	Antimicrobial	Dose and Route	Comments
group A β-hemolytic streptococci in patient with history of rheumatic fever	benzathine penicillin penicillin V sulfadiazine	1.2 mega U IM monthly 200,000 U P.O., b.i.d. daily 1 g P.O., daily	Benzathine penicillin most reliable. Prophylaxis continued to age 35 unless close contact with children continues –eg, school teacher, late parent.
group B streptococci in newborns	penicillin G	20,000 U/kg at birth	Prevents colonization and may prevent infection. However, may increase other gram-negative neonatal infection.
gonococcal ophthalmia in newborns	ceftriaxone	20-50 mg/kg x 1 dose	One dose effectively treats; eyedrops not needed.
chlamydial conjunctivitis in newborns	erythromycin, 0.5% ophthalmic ointment	one application at birth	Tetracycline, 1% ophthalmic ointment may be somewhat less effective.

3. Prevents colonization of surgically placed foreign body (hip prosthesis, artificial heart valve).
4. Protects individuals susceptible to reactivation of infection by virtue of medication or therapy (eg, patients with positive tuberculin tests on corticosteroids).
5. Protects patients with biologic propensity to develop bacterial complications (eg, patients with a history of rheumatic fever).
6. Protects patients prone to develop infection by virtue of immunologic structure (a) asplenic individuals; (b) agammaglobulinemic individuals; (c) women with recurrent urinary tract infections.

Bacterial Pathogen	Antimicrobial	Dose and Route	Comments
N meningitidis in crowded household or epidemic circumstances	ceftriaxone	250 mg IM x 1 dose (child <15 yr: 125 mg IM x 1 dose)	Variable and unreliable sensitivity to sulfa.
	ciprofloxacin	adults: 500 mg/d x 1 dose	
	rifampin*	adults: 600 mg P.O. b.i.d. x 2 days children: over 1 mo, 10 mg/kg b.i.d. x 2 d Under 1 month, 5 mg/kg b.i.d. x 2 d	Ciprofloxacin and rifampin not recommended in pregnancy. With rifampin, urine and tears may turn orange; may affect contact lenses.
H influenzae	rifampin*	20 mg/kg/d x 4 d (children) 600 mg/d P.O. x 4 d (adults)	May prevent spread in families and in day-care centers. Not to be used in pregnant women.
N gonorrhoeae	procaine penicillin G + probenecid	4.8 mega U IM x 1 1 g P.O. simultaneously	Penicillin resistance is increasing. Check VDRL.
	spectinomycin**	2 g IM x 1	

*Maximal dose is 600 mg/d P.O. for children.
**For penicillin-resistant strains.

continued on next page

Prophylactic Antibiotics *(continued)*

Surgical Usage

For preoperative surgical prophylaxis, dose should ideally be given 1 to 2 h preoperatively and, depending on pharmacokinetics, once intraoperatively, if necessary.

Disadvantages

1. Toxic and hypersensitivity reactions to the antibiotics; 2. Superinfection–often with more resistant organisms; 3. Alteration of ecology of hospital flora–select more resistant; 4. May encourage poor technique–hygienic and surgical.

Prophylaxis in Medical Situations *(continued)*

Bacterial Pathogen	Antimicrobial	Dose and Route	Comments
syphilis	benzathine penicillin	2.4 mega U IM x 1	Check VDRL later of contacts.
*M tuberculosis**	isoniazid	300 mg P.O., q.d. 6 mo-1 yr	a) Recent skin-test converters; b) High-level exposure, especially young children; c) Corticosteroid treatment with known positive skin test; d) Skin test (+) old chest lesion; e) PPD + less than 25-35 yr of age; f) Household contacts
Shigella in crowded, closed institutions	TMP/SMX**	TMP: 5 mg/kg b.i.d. SMX: 25 mg/kg b.i.d.	To stop outbreak. Quinolones, except in children, may have a role.
E coli in recurrent UTI	TMP/SMX or nitrofurantoin	1 tablet h.s.	Take postcoitus, or 3 times a week for 6 mo.

*See guidelines of American Thoracic Society *Am Rev Respir Dis* 1986;134: 355-363, and CDC recommendations *MMWR* 1990;39:RR-8 and *MMWR* 1993; 42:RR-7 for further explanation.

**Resistant strains have been reported from outside the United States.

Patterns of prophylaxis

1. Local, topical–thermal burns, aerosol, respiratory tract; 2. Systemic, before surgical procedure–heart, hip; 3. Meningococci, exposure to syphilis, recurrent urinary tract infection after coitus, rheumatic fever. Antibiotic prophylaxis not effective for viral URI, coma, cardiac failure, shock, cardiac catheterization.

Note: Because these recommendations are constantly changing, it is advised that the latest recommendations be used and that this text serve only as a guide.

Prophylaxis in Surgical Situations*

Procedure	Drug**	Dose	Comments
biliary tract	cephalosporin	1 g on call to OR, then 1-2 more doses that day	Older obese, diabetic patients with history of previous infections. History of obstruction.
	cefuroxime	1.5 g ½ to 1 h before surgery	
CNS shunts for hydrocephalus	oxacillin or vancomycin	1 g 1 g	Only need 2-3 doses.
colon surgery	erythromycin P.O. + neomycin P.O. +	1 g, at 1 p.m., 2 p.m., and 11 p.m. day before surgery	Only if no obstruction. Metronidazole used in Europe.
	1-3 doses of either cefoxitin or cefotetan	1 g, as above	
total hip replacement	cephalosporin vancomycin	1 g on call to OR, + 2nd dose during procedure	
	cefuroxime	1.5 g ½ to 1 h before surgery	
vaginal hysterectomy	cephalosporin	1 g on call to OR, intraoperatively if necessary	cefotetan or cefuroxime may be used
abdominal hysterectomy	cephalosporin	1 g on call to OR	Some studies show efficacy over placebo.

*Cefazolin is the usual agent, however, long-acting agents (ie, ceftriaxone), when given preoperatively, may provide protection throughout the procedure.

**Parenteral route unless otherwise indicated.

continued on next page

Prophylactic Antibiotics *(continued)*

Prophylaxis in Surgical Situations* *(continued)*

Procedure	Drug**	Dose	Comments
head and neck surgery- (cutting mucosal planes)	cephalosporin	1 g on call to OR	OR patients with radical surgery (not tonsillectomy).
	cefuroxime	1.5 g ½ to 1 h before surgery	clindamycin* gentamicin may be used
vascular surgery (Dacron grafts)	oxacillin or nafcillin or cephalosporin or vancomycin	1 g on call to OR, then q 8 h x 1 d	Though incidence of infection is low, infection may be disastrous.
	cefuroxime	1.5 g ½ to 1 h before surgery	
gastroduodenal	cephalosporin	1 g/1 h preoperatively	When GI motility is decreased, hemorrhage, obstruction, gastric ulcer, or malignancy
	cefuroxime	1.5 g ½ to 1 h before surgery	

*Cefazolin is the usual agent, however, long-acting agents (ie, ceftriaxone), when given preoperatively, may provide protection throughout the procedure.

**Parenteral route unless otherwise indicated.

Prophylaxis for Cardiac Surgery*

Use a regimen that contains an antistaphylococcal agent because both *S aureus and S epidermidis* are important pathogens in cardiac surgery.

Patient	Antibiotic	Dose	Route
cardiac surgery candidate	cephalosporin cefazolin** cephalothin cefamandole oxacillin. In addition, gentamicin may be added. cefuroxime	Give 1-2 g 30 min before surgery and q 6 h (q 8 h for cefazolin) for 6 or 8 doses 1.5 mg/kg 30 min before surgery, then q 8 h for 6 doses 1.5 g 1/2 to 1 h preoperatively and then q 12 h for total of 6 g***	IV IM IV
coronary artery bypass surgery candidate	cefazolin ceftriaxone[†] cefuroxime***	1-2 g 30 min before surgery and then q 8 h for 6 to 8 doses 1 g 1 h preoperatively; one dose appears effective 1.5 g 1/2 to 1 h preoperatively and then q 12 h for total of 6 g	IV IM IV IV

* *Although a variety of regimens is recommended by experts, patients may develop bacterial endocarditis even after receiving appropriate coverage. Since these recommendations are constantly changing, it is advised that the latest recommendations be used and that this text serve only as a guide.*

** Cefazolin has been proven to be an effective cephalosporin.

*** Please note that the dosage of cefuroxime is unique among the cephalosporins.

† Do not mix in same syringe with other agents or in same IV infusion with other agents; ceftriaxone solutions should not be physically mixed with other antimicrobial drugs because of possible incompatibility.

Prophylactic Antibiotics
(continued)

Prophylaxis for Dental Procedures and Surgical Procedures of the Upper Respiratory Tract*

Procedures

1. All dental procedures that are likely to result in gingival bleeding.
2. All surgery or instrumentation of the respiratory tract, such as tonsillectomy, adenoidectomy, bronchoscopy, and other surgical procedures of the upper respiratory tract involving disruption of the respiratory mucosa.

Special Considerations

For those patients receiving continuous oral penicillin for secondary prevention of rheumatic fever, alpha-hemolytic streptococci (which are relatively resistant to penicillin and occasionally found in the oral cavity). While it is likely that the doses of penicillin recommended are sufficient to control

Prophylaxis for Dental Procedures and Surgical Procedures of the Upper Respiratory Tract*

Condition	Patient/ Adults	Antibiotic Regimen	Dose
congenital heart disease rheumatic heart disease acquired valvular heart disease hypertrophic subaortic stenosis mitral valve prolapse with insufficiency prosthetic heart valve	adults not allergic to penicillin	ampicillin	2 g
		amoxicillin	2 g
	adults allergic to penicillin	vancomycin** or erythromycin • ethylsuccinate • stearate	1 g 1g 800 mg 1 g
		clindamycin	600 mg
prosthetic heart valve patients at high risk patients who cannot take oral medications	adults not allergic to penicillin	ampicillin gentamicin	2 g 1.5 mg/kg (not to exceed 80 mg)
	adults allergic to penicillin	vancomycin clindamycin	1 g 600 mg

*Recommendations by the American Heart Association, *JAMA* 1990:2919-2922.

**Considered to be at high risk.

Note: Although a variety of regimens is recommended by experts, patients may develop bacterial endocarditis even after receiving appropriate coverage. Since these recommendations are constantly changing, it is advised that the latest recommendations be used and that this text serve only as a guide.

these organisms, the physician or dentist may choose oral erythromycin.

In unusual circumstances or in the case of delayed healing, it may be prudent to provide additional doses of antibiotics even though available data suggest that bacteremia rarely persists longer than 15 minutes after the procedure.

Some patients with a prosthetic heart valve, in whom a high level of oral health is being maintained, may be offered oral antibiotic prophylaxis for routine dental procedures. However, parenteral antibiotics are recommended for patients with prosthetic valves who require extensive dental procedures, especially extractions, or oral or gingival surgical procedures.

In patients with significantly compromised renal function, it may be necessary to modify the dose of antibiotics used.

Route	Time Before Procedure (min)	Follow-up Antibiotic	Follow-up Dose*	Frequency
IM IV	30	ampicillin or amoxicillin	1 g IV 1.5 g P.O.	q 6 h 1 dose
P.O.	60	amoxicillin	1.5 g	q 6 h 1 dose
IV	administered over 1 h, beginning 1 h before			
P.O.	120	either one	½ dose P.O.	q 6 h 1 dose
P.O. IV	60 30	clindamycin clindamycin	150 mg P.O. 150 mg P.O. or IV	q 6 h 1 dose q 6 h 1 dose
IM, IV IM, IV	30	amoxicillin oral or repeat parenteral regimen	1.5 g	q 8 h 1 dose q 8 h 1 dose
IV	administered over 1 h, beginning 1 h before			

*Follow-up pediatric dose is one half original dose.

continued on next page

Prophylactic Antibiotics *(continued)*

Prophylaxis for Dental Procedures and Surgical Procedures of the Upper Respiratory Tract *(continued)*

Condition	Patient/ Children*	Antibiotic Regimen	Dose
congenital heart disease rheumatic heart disease acquired valvular heart disease hypertrophic subaortic stenosis mitral valve prolapse, insufficiency prosthetic heart valve	children not allergic to penicillin	amoxicillin clindamycin	amoxicillin dose for children: 50 mg/kg or amoxicillin doses for children*: <15 kg (33 lb) 750 mg 15-30 kg (33-66 lb) 1,500 mg >30 kg (66 lb) 3 g 10 mg/kg
	children allergic to penicillin	vancomycin** or erythromycin • ethylsuccinate • or stearate	20 mg/kg 20 mg/kg
prosthetic heart valves patients at high risk	children not allergic to penicillin	ampicillin gentamicin	50 mg/kg 2 mg/kg
	children allergic to penicillin	vancomycin**	20 mg/kg

* Doses for children not to exceed recommendations for adults for single 24-hour period.

** For vancomycin, the total dose for children should not exceed total adult dose.

Note: Although a variety of regimens is recommended by experts, patients may develop bacterial endocarditis even after receiving appropriate coverage. Since these recommendations are constantly changing, it is advised that the latest recommendations be used and that this text serve only as a guide.

Route	Time Before Procedure (min)	Follow-up Antibiotic	Follow-up Dose*	Frequency
P.O.	60	amoxicillin	1/2 dose	6 h later 1 dose
IV or P.O.	30 (IV) 60 (P.O.)	clindamycin	1/2 dose	6 h later 1 dose
IV	administered over 1 h, beginning 1 h before			
P.O.	120	erythromycin	10 mg/kg	q 6 h 1 dose
IM, IV	30	ampicillin	<60 lb 1/2 adult dosage	q 6 h 1 dose
IM, IV			P.O. or repeat parenteral regimen	q 8 h 1 dose
IV	60			

*Follow-up pediatric dose is one half original dose.

Prophylactic Antibiotics *(continued)*

Prophylaxis for Gastrointestinal and Genitourinary Surgery and Instrumentation

In patients with significantly compromised renal function, it may be necessary to modify the dose of antibiotics used. Some of these doses may exceed manufacturer's recommendations for a 24-hour period. However, since they are only recommended for a 24-hour period in most cases, it is unlikely that toxicity will occur.

Prophylaxis for Gastrointestinal and Genitourinary Surgery and Instrumentation

Patient	Antibiotic	Dose
adults and children* *not* allergic to penicillin	ampicillin +	2 g for adults 50 mg/kg for children (not to exceed 2 g)
	gentamicin	1.5 mg/kg for adults (not to exceed 120 mg 2 mg/kg for children)
allergic to penicillin	vancomycin +	1 g for adults, 20 mg/kg up to 1 g for children
	gentamicin	1.5 mg/kg (not to exceed 80 mg) for adults 2 mg/kg for children
oral regimen for minor or repetitive procedures in low-risk patients	*not* allergic to penicillin: amoxicillin	2 g for adults 50 mg/kg for children

*Children's dosage must not exceed maximum adult dosages.

During prolonged procedures, or in the case of delayed healing, it may be necessary to provide additional doses of antibiotics. For brief outpatient procedures, such as uncomplicated catheterization of the bladder, one dose may be sufficient.

Route	Comments
IM, IV IM, IV	Give initial doses 1/2 h before procedure; then ampicillin 1 g IM/IV or amoxicillin 1 g orally 6 h later
IV IM, IV	A single dose of these antibiotics should be given slowly and completed within 30 min of starting the procedure; the same dose may be repeated once in 8 h.
P.O.	Initial dose: 1 h before procedure, then 6 h later, 1/2 of dose

18

Index

B

C

D

E

F

G

H

I

M

N

O

P

Q

R

S

U

V

NOTES

NOTES

NOTES